W9-CEY-457

The VIEW from the WRONG SIDE of the DAY

A Story About Nursing, PTSD And Other Shenanigans

T. C. RANDALL

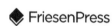 FriesenPress

Suite 300 - 990 Fort St
Victoria, BC, V8V 3K2
Canada

www.friesenpress.com

Copyright © 2020 by T. C. Randall
First Edition — 2020

All rights reserved.

No part of this publication may be reproduced in any form, or by any means, electronic or mechanical, including photocopying, recording, or any information browsing, storage, or retrieval system, without permission in writing from FriesenPress.

ISBN
978-1-5255-7002-5 (Hardcover)
978-1-5255-7003-2 (Paperback)
978-1-5255-7004-9 (eBook)

1. HEALTH & FITNESS, WORK-RELATED HEALTH

Distributed to the trade by The Ingram Book Company

To Tanya and Kevin, wherever you might be

FOREWORD

I would like to start with some advice. For those of you who are contemplating the purchase of this book, it would be wise at this point to pause and reflect upon your reasons for doing so. This is not a book about nursing, as such. Rather, it is a book about nurses, and about one nurse in particular (that would be me). If you are expecting humorous anecdotes about strange objects found in various body orifices or salacious tales of shenanigans gone awry, then this is probably not the book for you. You should, however, buy it anyway. I need the money.

This is a book about how I came to be a nurse, and the experiences I have had during that journey. It is also a book about my various adventures since becoming a nurse. In particular, I want to share with you the events of the last few years, as these have had a significant impact on my life. This is not to say that I won't have some colorful tales to tell, but those tales will be more about how they have impacted me and my co-workers. In truth, I'm not a big fan of war stories.

In those instances where I do discuss patients, I have changed certain details or combined details from several patients. Sometimes, I have purposely left the details vague. This is done to protect patient confidentiality. Every time I do discuss patients, it is strictly because of how important the events are to my own development as a nurse. If you happen upon a story that sounds like something you have personally experienced, I can assure you that this is purely coincidental.

I am writing this book in the hopes that other nurses might read these pages and see parts of their own stories. (It can't just be me, can it?) It is also my hope that they may see reflections of their own struggles, so that they will not feel as isolated and alone. There really is strength in numbers.

I want to stress the point that this book is not meant as a criticism of any individual. It is not even meant as a criticism of any particular institution. The purpose is to shine a light on certain systemic inadequacies, so that they might be addressed and altered in the future. There are many events that I have experienced over the last four years that should never happen to anyone ever again. In order to bring about change, we must first have an open and honest dialog. I am hoping that this book will at least get the conversation going.

I should also stress that the words in these pages are based on my own opinions. As all humans do, I have interpreted events based upon my own observations, as well as my own personal biases. I humbly apologize if I have gotten anything wrong or if I have unjustly maligned anyone. That is completely unintentional.

Far from being negative, it is my hope that these words will serve as both inspiration and warning; though if I happen to get a few laughs along the way, I will not be disappointed.

While reading, you may find the flow difficult to follow at times. I tend to jump around a little, switching from one subject to another and then back again. I can also ramble at times. I have left it this way on purpose. I think that, by retaining *some* of the original chaos in my writing, it will provide a small amount of insight into how my mind functions at present. I used to be hyper-organized. Now, my thoughts tend to be scattered. Welcome to my brain.

Don't be overly concerned if you are not a nurse, for there may be something within these pages for you as well. Some of the specific references might not resonate, but I believe the overall theme is one that many people have been through in their own lives. Who hasn't run up against bureaucracies, bad decisions by management, and stress at work? I think this is especially true for those who hold jobs in fields similar to mine. There are many others who are exposed to horrific events daily, such as doctors, police officers, firefighters, paramedics, and those serving in the military. Parts of my story will be very familiar to these people, unfortunately.

If you love someone who is employed in one of these professions, there might also be some benefit for you. This book will give you a glimpse into our daily lives. Perhaps it will also give you some insight into why we are always so screwed in the head. I separated from my wife early in my nursing career because, as she stated, I never talked to her. She subsequently attended nursing school herself. I can remember vividly the day she came to me and said, "Ok, now I get it."

Whatever your background, I hope that you find within these pages something that is meaningful to you personally. At the very least, I hope you find something that makes you laugh a little. Take heed, however. We nurses have a rather *unique* sense of humor.

There are many people that have impacted my life over the years, and I have included some of them within these pages. I have not used any names, but some may still recognize themselves by the events that I describe. For those who do, please forgive me if I have gotten any of the details wrong. My memory is not what it once was (I'm getting old). If I did not mention you, please know that this is not meant as a slight. In no way is this meant to imply that you are any less important to me. If I mentioned every single person or event from the last twenty years, this book would be very long.

I also must give a huge thank-you to those who have aided me in this project. Over the last few months, several of my friends have had to read over my many drafts. They have had to endure my incessant nagging, and it is a wonder that none of them has tried to shoot me yet. Without these people, this book would probably never have been written. At the very least, it would not have been written well. The grammar alone would most likely have driven every one of my readers insane. Thank you so much, all of you.

There is one other thing that I should mention so that certain passages make sense. There is an organization that is meant to support injured workers. I would really prefer if they didn't sue me, so I shall be referring to them in code. I shall call them NATH (Not All That Helpful). There is a section of NATH that I have been dealing with for the last few months. I will call them ALMH (A Little More Helpful).

I suppose, in closing, that I should say something about the title of this book. Some of you might be wondering where it came from and what the hell it means. If you are not at all curious, indulge me anyway. It came to me once at the end of a night shift. I was outside just as the sun began to rise, and it occurred to me how strange it was to be seeing a new day dawn when I had not been to sleep yet. Being very tired, I thought to myself, "This is just the wrong side of the day." As soon as those words came to me, I knew that I just had to use them as the title of a book someday. Now I have.

IN THE BEGINNING

Now would be a good time to introduce myself. My name is T. C. Randall (it's really not, but that's the way it's going to be). I was born somewhere and, up until this point, I have also done some stuff. All in all, I would say that my life has been an interesting one. As you may have already gathered, however, I am not going to be including any stories from my past within these pages.

First off, I do not believe that my history really pertains to this particular story. I have deliberately focused on one specific period in my life because of its importance to me personally. Second, I am hoping to retain some sense of mystery about myself. Perhaps the most important reason, however, is that I might just be able to finagle another book out of this deal. That would depend, of course, on how well this book does. Always plan for the long game, I say.

I began my career as an emergency room nurse sixteen years ago, though two of those years were as a student nurse. Apparently, the average life span for an ER nurse is eight years, so I stayed well past my due date. As a result, I have been out of work for two years now due to post-traumatic stress. The following story is meant to help you understand how I got here.

My tale begins way back in the mid-1990s. I know. I just stated that I would not be including past events. It is pertinent, however, so bear with me here. I was working minimum wage jobs at the time (flipping burgers) and was feeling more than a little dissatisfied with my life. The city I was living in was very expensive, so even my crappy little studio apartment was more than I could afford. I cannot even say that I was living paycheck to paycheck because that would imply my paychecks were covering my expenses. They were not, and I was falling further and further behind. It was time to try something new.

I can't remember exactly what it was that inspired me, but I hit upon the idea of becoming a paramedic. I loved the idea of helping people, especially when they need that help the most. Also, I really wanted to do something with my life that had meaning. I was good at what I did, but I seriously doubt that anyone ever found one of my burgers to be life-altering. Besides, I needed more out of life. I was in desperate need of something more fulfilling. I was also tired of being broke *all the time*! The prospect of setting off on a new path was very appealing to me.

I signed up for a specialized first aid course, which was the prerequisite for becoming a paramedic at the time. Taking that course was an amazing experience. I had found myself. There is a certain feeling that one gets upon experiencing one's true calling for the first time. It's like a rush of enthusiasm, and everything just seems to click into place. It was simply astounding. Without a doubt, this was the first time in my life that I had truly put 100 percent of myself into anything. The most appealing part of first aid is that there is an order to it, like a dance. Details must be recognized and acted upon in a concise pattern and in a timely manner. Apparently, I thrive in this type of environment.

I also found that I possess almost no sense of squeamishness whatsoever. Almost nothing fazes me. I am the type of person who could see someone's insides spilling out and still eat my lunch right afterwards. This is a good trait to have in the medical field, as you can imagine.

Now, I did say *almost*. I will admit to one weakness. For some reason, eyeballs really freak me out. They are just so gross and squishy. During the first aid course, we would practice on each other, fixing simulated injuries. One of my classmates had to practice treating me for an eye injury. I can remember feeling very sorry for the poor guy. He did his best, but, in half an hour, he did not even get close to my eyes. My head was weaving back and forth like some sort of bobblehead figurine on someone's dashboard. In fact, I am sure that I came very close to kicking him a few times. Other people's eyes are no better. In fact, just writing this is sending shivers up and down my spine. That is why I still wear glasses. There is no way in hell that I would ever be able to wear contact lenses, simply because I would never be able to actually get them in.

The part of the course I most enjoyed was learning about anatomy. As this was just a first aid course, it was very rudimentary. Still, it piqued my curiosity, and that has never faded. I find it fascinating just how everything in our bodies fits together and how everything works as a unit to keep us alive. Every system interacts with every other system. My greatest strength throughout my career has been that I am never satisfied just knowing what I must do. I also have an insatiable need to understand why.

After the course was over, I hit a snag. This course had been designed for workplace injuries. It wasn't enough to just pass the course; we were required to take a test at the local NATH office in order to receive our certification. This entailed running through several scenarios to ensure that we had *some* idea of what we were doing. I had performed quite well during the course itself, so I did not foresee any problems. Of course, when test day came, I awoke with a high fever and a head that felt about three sizes too large. To say that I felt like crap would be understating it. As I had already paid the non-refundable exam fee, I decided to soldier on and proceeded to the testing facility.

Now, to understand what happened next, I must clarify something. One of the main criteria for the test was time. In a seriously injured casualty, we were given fifteen minutes to identify and treat any life-threatening injuries and to get the patient all packed up and into the ambulance. Though I felt pretty dopey by this point, I had practiced my little heart out in the days prior. As a result, my times had been well under the limit. Even sick, I was reasonably certain that I could still meet the challenge in the time allotted.

When my turn came to run through a scenario, I was slower than I had been previously. However, I still managed to do everything that had been required, just as my fifteen minutes came to an end. I looked up and could see that the tester was busy watching another student. This was when I made a critical mistake. Instead of continuing, which is what I was supposed to do, I stopped and waited for her to look my way. I had assumed that she would need to see what I had completed before I proceeded any further. However, when she did turn my way a few moments later, the conversation that ensued went like this:

Tester: "What should you be doing now?"

Me: "Loading him into the ambulance."

Tester: "So why aren't you doing that?"

Me: "Because I was waiting for you."

She failed me for going over the time limit! I can't recall ever feeling that defeated before. It seemed to me a great injustice. I had loved everything about the course I had taken. This felt like my destiny. Now, I had failed. Not because I had done anything wrong, but because of a simple misunderstanding. I could have given it all up right there. Luckily, my instructor talked me into taking the exam again, even though it meant spending another $100, which I really didn't have at the time. I am glad that I never took the failure to heart, or it could have seriously damaged my confidence. As it was, I knew that I had not made any mistakes, and that the failure was due to circumstance. The second time I took the exam, I passed easily. If I had not returned for another try, my life might have turned out very differently.

Two years later, I had to go back to NATH and renew my certification. I ended up with the same tester again, but I don't think that she recognized me. The poor woman must have wondered why I kept glaring at her throughout the day. I easily passed that test, in case you were wondering. Take that Ms. Examiner!

Then came another snag, though I had known about this one ahead of time. See, at this point, I had lived most of my life in big cities. In most cities, public transportation is both more affordable and easier than driving. That, coupled with my relative poverty, meant that I had never bothered to get my driver's license. Unfortunately, if you are going to work for the ambulance service, they prefer if you are able to drive said ambulances. Those puppies don't drive themselves. This, of course, requires a driver's license. And not just any old license either. No, paramedics need a special type of license. This left me with a bit of a dilemma. Here I had the first aid training, but the driving would require me to get a regular license. I would then have to wait a further two years before I could get the special license.

While I waited, I needed something else to do. I also needed money so that I could afford to get my regular driver's license. Luckily, my first aid certificate also enabled me to work as a first aid attendant in construction, which I did for the next year. I must admit, this experience was a bit of a letdown. Apparently, the classroom and real life tend to differ, so perhaps my expectations were a little high. I thought I was going to be a lifesaver, sitting in my first aid room healing the injured. I thought that I was going to be some sort of hero. You know, like on TV. Alas, no such noble pursuit awaited me. It turns out that construction companies don't like having people just sitting around. I was put to work. And as a first aid person, that meant I mostly had to do grunt work. Now, I am in no way disparaging grunt work. I have worked hard my entire adult life, and grunt work is both necessary and honorable in my books. It just wasn't what I had been expecting.

Most of my days consisted of wandering around picking up and appropriately disposing of all the scraps that the various trades had left behind: pieces of wood, scraps of metal, old wiring, etc. As a first aid attendant, the only restriction was that I could not do any job I could not leave immediately, in case an emergency occurred. I had to be ready to respond at a moment's notice. Because of this restriction, most of the jobs on site were off limits. All that really remained was garbage duty.

On one site, I was also given the task of putting up all the safety barriers. It was a new apartment building, and all that had been erected so far was the concrete outer structure. As a result, all the balconies had to have wooden frames across the openings so that no one would fall. That was actually a fun job. It gave me something to do that felt important and was also in line with my role of keeping people safe. I did, however, slip and drop one of the two-by-fours once. The people below were not happy, and I had come very close to creating my first serious casualty all on my own. My credibility suffered a bit that day, I think.

During this period, I began to realize just how idiotic most of my fellow men are. Sorry guys, but it's true. For some reason, we, as a gender, are completely oblivious to any sense of self-preservation. Seeing what I saw on every site I worked at, it is a wonder that anyone survived. For instance, I would often see roofers wandering about without harnesses on, several stories above the ground. I recall one individual who was actually leaning out over the side of the building, hammering a nail. He was eight stories up and very precariously balanced, I must add. I recall thinking to myself that if he had fallen, I would not have needed to bring my first aid gear at all. A mop and bucket would have sufficed.

On one occasion, I was sent to another site that already had a first aid attendant. When I asked him why they had needed me there, he told me that he would sometimes faint at the sight of blood. This was the guy who was supposed to be responsible for people's safety!

Now, don't get me wrong. There were some definite plusses to the job as well. For starters, as a first aid attendant, I did enjoy a certain amount of authority on the sites where I worked. I was often in charge of site safety. This gave me some measure of power when it came to ensuring that regulations were being adhered to. Walking around, I would often see the tradespeople scrambling around to replace their hard hats on their heads when they saw me coming.

I also had the final say on all things medical. Once, I remember arguing with one of my bosses. He was put out because I would not let a worker return to his job for fifteen minutes after he had been stung by a wasp. He had never been stung before, and I needed to watch for an allergic reaction. The boss was not happy at the delay, but I won the argument.

...

About a year later, I moved to a small town. Unfortunately, it turned out that none of the local construction companies required first aid attendants. I should say, rather, that most companies trained their foremen as first aid people. Being a small town, the work wasn't as steady for construction companies as it had been in the city, so this was a cost cutting measure. Combining the two roles meant that there was one less person to pay.

Around this time, the rules for becoming a paramedic were changed. In the past, once a person had their first aid certificate, he or she could apply to become a paramedic. Once hired, the candidate would then be sent to take the more advanced paramedic course. In order to save money, this was changed so that anyone wanting to become a paramedic would also have to pay for the advanced course themselves. This essentially put becoming a paramedic out of my reach, at least for the time being. I might have been able to afford the course itself, but there was no way I could manage without pay for that amount of time. Also, I still had no driver's license. Basically, I was left with no alternative but to return to minimum wage jobs for a while.

In order to keep my skills up, I started to do some volunteer work. I signed up with an organization that would do first aid for various local events. This allowed me to keep in practice. It also provided me with some real-world experiences. At the events we covered, most injuries were limited to scrapes and bruises. There were lots of bee stings during the summer months or the occasional heat stroke. Simple things.

We also trained together every week, which further enhanced my skills. A few of the members had been volunteering for a long time, and they proved to be a great source of information.

My participation in this organization also led me to get work as a first aid instructor. It was very part-time, of course, but I found that I immensely enjoyed teaching. I also found that I have a real aptitude for it. I possess a skill for taking complex ideas and translating them into simple explanations. As I tend to think in metaphors anyway, I am able to convey difficult concepts by relating them to everyday occurrences. For instance, I always compare the kidneys to a spaghetti strainer as they work in a somewhat similar fashion. People seem to get it, and that gives me a feeling of real accomplishment.

One huge benefit to these experiences was that I began to develop a real sense of confidence. Not only were my skills improving, but I was also gaining some experience in dealing with actual people. This has proved invaluable throughout my career, simply because it is something that I struggle with. I am a natural introvert, so in the beginning my people skills were in desperate need of some improvements. By the time I signed up for nursing school, I had learned how to develop a rapport with my patients and to project a sense of competence.

As you can imagine, in an emergency, people need to feel that the person looking after them knows what they are doing. I could be the best first aid person/paramedic/nurse/doctor on the planet and it matters not one iota if the patient doesn't believe it. I owe a great deal of my talent as a nurse to this period of time. For the opportunities I was given over those few years, I am truly grateful.

I am sure that many of you are wishing I would just get on with it already. Well, you are in luck.

It was at this point that I decided to go back to school and become a nurse. How I came to this decision is a strange but fascinating tale. I was watching an episode of *ER*, and Julianna Margulies' character (Carol Hathaway) had a patient who was dying. There was nothing she could do to help him, so instead she just sat with him while he died. It was an extremely emotional episode for me. In fact, it remains one of the few times I have ever seen the power of nursing accurately portrayed on TV. The entire process that they shared was so intimate and extraordinary.

In the medical field, it can be very easy to get sucked in by the clinical sometimes. What appealed to me most about nursing was that I would also be able to tap into my compassion. I would be able to forge real connections with patients, rather than simply being able to *fix* them. I was completely hooked from that moment on. I also knew exactly where I wanted to work when I was done. The emergency room seemed like the place for me. I was really drawn to the idea of helping people at their most vulnerable. I also must admit to liking the excitement.

Still, my new career path did not come about overnight. The biggest obstacle, I felt, was my age. I was not exactly a young man, even at that point. I wasn't all that old either—just older than most of the people who attend college. Therefore, going back to school for four years seemed a daunting prospect at first. It would also require another two years of study before I could even apply to the program, making it six years in total. The first year, I had to upgrade some of my high school courses. Apparently, there is a time limit for how long my previous educational accomplishments were considered valid. I believe that the cutoff was ten years. In the second year, I had to take prerequisite courses at the university level: biology, English, and an elective (I chose to take psychology).

I believe I stalled for the better part of a year as I hemmed and hawed. The age factor was difficult to overcome for me. The funny thing about stalling is that you don't tend to get anywhere. Fortunately, I had an epiphany. I realized that in six years' time, it was still going to be six years later. I could either be right where I was or doing something new and exciting. Time doesn't care, it just keeps moving forward. For those of you out there contemplating making a similar change, but feel you are too old, I will say it again: in six years' time, it will still be six years later.

As I found out later, many male nurses actually start later in life anyway. It's almost always a second or third career for us. To be honest, I don't remember it even being brought up as an option when I was growing up. There were no role models. Everyone just knew that nurses were women. The only time that I can recall seeing a male nurse on TV was an episode of M*A*S*H. Once, just after starting the nursing program, I had someone ask me if I was even allowed to be a nurse. The irony of this is that, up until recent times, nursing was mostly a male profession. The first nurses were monks. During the middle ages, nuns began to take on nursing duties in some hospitals, while monks remained as nurses on the battlefield. It wasn't until Florence Nightingale came along that women really took over the profession. It is a real shame because I think that men can be great nurses. Unfortunately, there's such a stereotype present that many men will not even consider nursing as a career. Female doctors must face similar challenges, I imagine. I have been called doctor more times than I can count at work, and I'm sure that many of the female doctors are just as sick and tired of being called nurse.

Of course, in the end, I did make the decision to enroll in the nursing program. It was the best decision of my life.

The first year, as I mentioned, I was forced to redo some of the high school courses. I ended up taking chemistry, biology, and math. A moment of bragging here. I was excused from having to redo English because, apparently, I received one of the highest scores that they had ever seen on the reading comprehension test. I know, you are all very impressed.

Let me tell you, education really is wasted on the young. Back in high school, I believe that most of my time was spent hanging around outside in the smoking area. It certainly wasn't spent in class. In truth, school just bored me as a youth. Returning as an adult learner, however, was a totally different experience. By choosing to be there, I felt invested in the process. I actually paid attention —and, boy, had I missed out. That year, I gained a true appreciation for the entire learning process.

By far, my favorite course that first year was chemistry. It appealed to me for two reasons. First, it was all math. I have a bit of a math brain, so the calculations came easily to me. Second, I also have a very high aptitude for three-dimensional thinking. As a result, I could easily picture molecules in my head, turning them over to see how they fit together. They were like three-dimensional jigsaw puzzles in my mind. That absolutely fascinated me.

Our chemistry teacher was great as well. He looked like the epitome of a mad scientist. I'm not sure he even owned a hairbrush. Yet, he taught with a passion that inspired us. It was obvious that he loved his work, and I know that I got caught up in his enthusiasm as a result. We all did. He remains one of my favorite teachers ever.

Math was more of a struggle. Not because it was difficult, but because it wasn't. The only reason that I was forced to retake the math courses in the first place was because it had been so long ago that I had taken them. I had forgotten a great deal, so I had scored low on the math placement test. That is very embarrassing for a math brain like me. However, it was very easy to pick up again. I can't remember if I had to repeat two years or three. I just remember what a major slog it was. We also didn't have any classroom time for the courses, so it was all self-directed learning. I'm a pretty clever guy; disciplined, not so much. Without having someone to drive me on, it was very hard to remain focused and get the work done.

I don't remember much from biology at all, to be honest. I remember finding it interesting at the time, but I think a lot of it was about plants. Not being relevant to my career path, none of it really stuck in my memory. The only part that I do remember was learning about genetics, which I did find fascinating. Unfortunately, it seemed to involve a great deal of learning about peas, so....

The highlight of that first year had absolutely nothing to do with school. At the beginning of the summer break, I made a trip down to the big city to see one of my favorite bands play. Several friends came with, and someone could have followed us around by the trail of empty Jack Daniel's bottles we had left behind like breadcrumbs. I am not even sure how we survived. My blood was probably 50 percent alcohol by the end of the night. The worst part was that the singer appeared to be even more intoxicated than we were, I think. He couldn't even remember the lyrics and the band had to cover for him. I say that "I think" that's what happened because it all remains just a little foggy. Still, I had not danced that hard in a long time. This was really my last big blow out. If I tried to do that now, at my present age, I would likely never recover.

The next day was very painful. That I can recall all too well. Every inch of my body was hurting, even my hair.

Anyway, enough about my adventures. On to the next year.

Once we had been accepted into the nursing program, we were required to take several courses as prerequisites. For starters, there was an anatomy course and an essay writing course. In addition, we had to complete three electives during the nursing program, one of which we had to take before starting. As I mentioned earlier, I chose psychology. Since the anatomy course counted as two credits (class and lab), that added up to four credits in total. I was told that this was a fairly standard course load for most students. If only I had listened.

For some bizarre reason, I also signed up for organic chemistry. At the time I had assumed that it would just be a continuation of the high school chemistry. I had enjoyed chemistry so much the previous year. I remember one of the administrative people had looked at my course selections with a wary eye. She had warned me against such a heavy course load, but I was determined to sign up anyway. Organic chemistry was an entirely different universe. It was far more difficult than I had been expecting. Also, the instructor spoke very quietly. Perhaps the course really wasn't that difficult, but I don't think I could hear a word the instructor said. In the end, it proved too much, and I was forced to drop the course.

Now, I would like to mention that my second year took place in 2001. I can remember walking to school one day (the college was up this great big hill), when a friend called to tell me that a plane had just hit the World Trade Center. Now, in my mind, I'm seeing a Cessna or some other small plane. Thinking that it had been an accident, I remember wondering how someone could possibly hit a building like that. Did the pilot not see this huge metal tower getting larger and larger in the window? It wasn't until lunch time that I actually saw a TV. I got quite a shock at that point. It had definitely *not* been an accident. I know that this has nothing at all to do with my story, but there are just certain events that stick with you forever. I am sure that anyone reading this who was alive that day knows exactly what I'm talking about.

Anyway, back to my story.

Apart from the chemistry, I really did enjoy my studies that year. The anatomy course we had to take was very in depth and comprehensive. Our instructor was also a retired RN so she got right down to what we needed to know and threw out all the rest. As a result, it was a fast paced and informative course. I loved every minute of it. This may sound strange, but I believe that my talent for three-dimensional thinking helped me a great deal during this course. It's not like chemistry, where I was able to see the molecules in my head. Yet, somehow, I found it very easy to understand anyway. It was as if I was better able to grasp how everything in our bodies is connected and how systems are able to interact with one another. The human body is simply another example of a three-dimensional jigsaw puzzle, just a great deal more complicated. That probably makes no sense at all, but it is the only way that I can describe my experience.

Of course, I loved my English course. I may be good at math but reading and writing are my most favorite activities ever. They are my true passion. I had written a great deal way back in high school, where I was quite well known for my storytelling. I even considered becoming a journalist at one point. Unfortunately, the course itself ended up being totally irrelevant to the nursing program. I am still not sure why this it was a prerequisite.

Psychology was also a favorite. In truth, it is a subject that I had always been curious about. I am truly fascinated by how the human mind works and how that translates into behavior. Deep down, I believe that we are all just the product of our past experiences.

I will also admit to a morbid fascination with the darker aspects of humanity. I have always felt a need to understand where such behaviors come from.

I include myself in that need to understand. Part of my fascination with psychology is in looking at my own behaviors and wondering where they come from. My therapist commented recently on my ability to look at myself with a certain clinical detachment, even as I go through the process as a patient. I believe self-reflection is a talent that is highly underutilized in today's society, and it shouldn't be. We all have parts of ourselves we don't like, and not one of us is perfect. Without self-reflection, there is no moving forward, and our lives become an endless cycle of doing the same dumb stuff over and over again. Without self-reflection, we can't learn or change. Sometimes we need to look deep into ourselves and just ask WTF?

Besides, without self-reflection this book would not exist.

WELCOME TO NURSING SCHOOL
(AKA THE GAPING JAWS OF HELL)

F irst off, thanks to those of you who have made it this far. Your tenacity is greatly appreciated. Now we can get to the part that relates directly to nursing.

Not many people realize this, but nursing is considered one of the toughest undergraduate degrees there is. Now, before anyone gets all riled up, I did say "one of." I know, there was that thing a few years ago. Many professions were posting about how Guinness World Records had officially recognized their program as the hardest. It was a hoax. Get over it. I also said undergraduate degree, so all of you doctors out there can calm down. I personally do believe it to be *the* toughest undergraduate degree, simply due to the volume of writing that is involved. We had several papers to write for each course, weekly journaling, tests, and several group projects to complete. Toward the end of each semester, I could easily be producing twenty typewritten pages a week. On top of that, there were also care plans to write up for all our patients. I would also do up handwritten index cards for every medication that I encountered. If nursing isn't the hardest program, this still represents an enormous amount of work.

I also need to mention our books. You can always tell who the first-year nursing students are (or any other first-year students, really) by the forklifts they have to bring with them on textbook day. Don't forget that, at this point in my life, I still didn't drive. So, there's me: I was trying to make my way home, down the big hill, with a twenty-foot-tall stack of books in my arms. I couldn't even see, so I had to resort to traffic noises as a mode of navigation, like some sort of weird sonar. If the traffic noises started to get louder, I had to veer to the right so that I didn't wander out onto the road.

There is also the fact that textbooks aren't like regular books. After all, students are a captive audience, so to speak. I can remember a meme I saw a few years ago. It showed a newspaper article, which outlined how someone had stolen twenty thousand dollars' worth of textbooks. Someone had cleverly written underneath, "I hope they recovered both of the books." This is not an exaggeration. That twenty-foot stack of books cost about the same as a new house. To this day, it remains my most expensive single purchase ever.

Before I could start the program, there was one more item that I needed to take care of. At the time, I was working in the worst restaurant ever. I mean, the staff was good, and the food was decent. The boss, however, was something of an idiot. He was so cheap that nothing was ever done properly. For instance, he tried to save money by never getting the vents in the kitchen cleaned. It did save him some money, until the fans seized up with grease and blew a hole in the roof. He ended up spending several thousand dollars on repairs, just to save a few bucks. That's the kind of place it was.

Anyway, I had informed the boss man that my school year was starting and that I would now only be able to work part-time on the weekends. On the Friday before I started classes, I was surprised to find that I had been scheduled for the full week instead. He had known for months what was happening, so it is not as if he had not had time to plan for this. I was so incredibly angry at him in that moment. I started my shift, but in the middle of lunch someone said the wrong thing to me (I can't even remember what the person said), and I walked out. The surprise on everyone's face as I headed for the door was priceless. I never went back there, other than to pick up my last paycheck.

. . .

On the first day of nursing school, I can remember feeling very excited. That was somewhat dampened when I arrived for my very first class and found out that it was in a portable. For those of you that don't know, a portable is a fancy word for a big metal box with no heat. There's also no sunlight to speak of. There are just a couple of tiny windows high up on the walls, just like the ones you see in old-style dungeons on the History Channel. And there are some of those awful seizure-inducing florescent lights on the ceiling that flicker constantly. Essentially, portables are how classrooms would be designed if they were constructed in hell.

As is probably the case in many university programs, we spent most of the first day introducing ourselves. We had to talk about our lives, and then we divided up into smaller groups and talked about ourselves some more. After an hour or so, we moved on to the next class and started the process all over again. We were also forced to participate in those awful communication games and team-building exercises. For introverts like me, this is akin to a serious form of torture. The UN needs to investigate this. I believe this went on for about a week. I wanted to bash my own head in with a hammer by the end of it.

In the first week we also received the assignment list for the semester, along with the due dates for each. That was quite the shock to the system. As I stated earlier, there is an enormous amount of writing in nursing school. Most of the written assignments in first year were all about self-reflection. We were expected to dig deep into our own psyches, and then spew forth whatever darkness we found lurking there. Essentially, the more we could write about what horrible people we were, the higher the grade we would receive. No one enjoys looking that closely at their deepest thoughts and feelings, let alone sharing them with the world. It was an emotionally grueling and time-consuming process—one that involved examining all of the nasty bits we would prefer to keep hidden, especially from ourselves. Unfortunately, this process is a necessary one for nurses. To know our patients, we must know ourselves first. Carrying around a whole lot of baggage gets in the way of that, so it has to be unloaded somehow.

At this point, I should probably admit that I was somewhat of a lazy student. I was literally the king of procrastination. In general, I preferred to write my assignments at the last possible second. This meant a lot of all-nighters. My saving grace was that I knew how to write fairly well. Often, I had most of the essay already written in my head, and I just had to get it down on paper. Unfortunately, I am also very bad at typing. (I have since improved. I must be one of the world's fastest one-finger typists now.) There were times when I seriously underestimated just how long an assignment would take me to type out. Hence the sleepless nights. Coffee and I began a serious relationship during this time, and I am happy to report that we are still going strong.

Earlier I mentioned that I did not find the prerequisite English class helpful. It is quite simple, really. In university level writing, it is not enough to state an opinion. You damn well better be able to back it up. This means that you have to do a great deal of research. The problem comes when choosing one of the four (that I know of) completely different ways of citing sources. Nursing is considered a science, so we used APA (American Psychological Association) citations. Our English class used MLA (Modern Language Association) citations. These two systems are somewhat different in how the citations are structured. As a result, my citations were a mess because I was already used to writing them a different way. In third year, I had to write a very long paper on nursing theory. The instructor informed me that she would have given me a perfect grade, if not for the fact that my APA was "not even at a beginner level." I could never figure out why. It wasn't until my ex was in nursing school that I began to understand some of the things I had been doing wrong. It would have been much more helpful to take an English course that had incorporated APA style instead.

...

Each year of nursing school was divided into three semesters. The fall semester ran from September to December. The winter semester from January to May. Then there was the spring semester that would take us till the end of June.

During our fall semester that first year, we were not allowed anywhere near a real patient. Probably for very good reason. Instead, we spent our time participating in a strange ritual called "lab". Here, we would practice basic nursing skills on each other or on mannequins. This, of course, had no bearing on actual nursing. For starters, the mannequins tended to be fairly compliant. They would patiently lay there while we gave them bed baths or practiced feeding them. They also tended to be on the thin side, which made them easy to move around and roll over. Real patients sometimes tend to be larger, especially those that are immobile, or bed bound. They also wriggle around a lot more. Often, the elderly patients with dementia will even attempt to bite us or punch us in the side of the head. Trying to give a real patient a bed bath is often more like trying to wrestle a full-grown grizzly bear that has been covered in Vaseline.

Our skills were basic in first year. We focused mostly on things like hygiene and how to properly mobilize patients (get them up and walking). There were also some basic assessment skills, like how to listen to a patient's chest. This meant actually using the stethoscopes we carried around with us. Until then, I had worn my stethoscope around as more of a "don't I look cool" statement. I'm hoping I'm not the only one who did this.

In case you are wondering, a new stethoscope costs about the same as my monthly car payment.

Hand washing was also a big part of first year. Apparently, we had all been doing it wrong for years. In health care, proper hand washing is a very important skill. I had never viewed it as an activity that one needed to practice, in all honesty. Yet, there is a definite technique to it. We had to make sure that we were getting into every nook and cranny. During first year, the correct response to any question was "wash my hands."

We also learned a lot about medications. Of course, all medications were new to us at this point, so each one had to be looked up and investigated. We would tirelessly research every medication we came across: how they were given, what side effects they had, what a correct dosage would be. We were also taught how to correctly give medications. There are checks that nurses go through with all medications to ensure that patients get what they are supposed to. When I went to school, we called these the "seven" rights: right medication, right patient, right dosage, right route (you cannot imagine the look a patient gets when they try to chew a suppository), right time, right reason, right documentation.

Unfortunately, these days I have become quite the expert on medications. That's because I am now taking most of them myself.

Back then, I imagine I took a long time to go through all of that. With practice it gets faster, fortunately. If it took me half the time now, I would still never get through it. Here's the thing, though. I still go through the same process with every medication I give. If I am unfamiliar with a medication, or if I haven't given it in a while, I will look it up for side effects, etc. That is one thing from nursing school that really sunk in. Because of this practice, I have only made three medication errors during my entire career.

At some point during our first year, we were also taught how to give injections. That was the best part of the entire year, if you ask me. I always tell patients that I became a nurse simply because they let me play with the sharp things. (Joking, of course. Well, maybe not entirely.)

...

During our third semester, we were sent off to extended care for our first patient experience. I have always wondered at the logic of this. Senior care is not easy. Yes, we are not going to cure them in the traditional medical sense, so they are not considered acute. However, every one of them had complex and intertwining medical conditions that we understood very little at that point in our education. To me, having the first-year nursing students look after vulnerable seniors speaks heavily to how little regard we hold for seniors in our society. It was as if they were seen as somewhat expendable, just in case we screwed something up. They say that the beginning of wisdom is realizing how much we don't know. I felt very wise that first year.

One thing that surprised me about long-term care was seeing how many of the patients had get well cards on their bedside tables or tacked up on their walls. I hope this doesn't sound crass, but there is really only one way out of extended care for patients. Having an over-developed sense of irony, the cards always struck me as just a little bit absurd.

I don't think that any nursing student ever forgets his or her first patient. Mine was a very kindly elderly gentleman. He was unable to stand without assistance, so he needed my help whenever he had to get out of bed. On my very first day, I needed to help him get dressed and ready for breakfast. I was attempting to lift him up off the bed, but for some reason I couldn't. He was stuck somehow. I looked down and one of his feet, twisted at a horrible angle, was trapped by the bed rail. To this day, I don't know how it didn't break with me tugging at him like I was. Even so, it still must have hurt a great deal. I still get shivers and a little tinge of guilt when I think about it. Luckily, he was very understanding. He accepted my apology and we moved on.

For the first week, we had one patient, and all we had to do was take care of their basic needs (such as getting them up for breakfast without injuring them). As the semester progressed, we added another patient, then another. We also added in more tasks, such as being responsible for their medications. It was a slow progression, with a great deal of supervision. Still, by the end of the semester, we were doing most of the work for our assigned patients.

One cherished memory from this time did not even involve one of my patients. I was walking down the hallway one day when I heard someone crying. When I investigated, I found one of the residents sitting in her wheelchair, weeping. She had very advanced dementia, and apparently this was quite common for her. When I entered the room, she grabbed my hand and just held it. Instead of pulling away, I sat down beside her and stayed there for about an hour. I am sure she had no idea who I was, but she still quieted right down. Just knowing that someone else was there seemed enough to reassure her. One of the things I most loved about nursing school was that we could sometimes spend more time just being with our patients. It's an aspect that I sorely miss as an RN. Unfortunately, there just isn't time anymore.

If there is one perception that I took with me from that first experience, it is just how much we have abandoned our senior population in this society. Let me be very clear here, this is in no way meant to disparage the staff because they performed to the very best of their abilities. Despite their best intentions, however, the care given was minimal. Because of understaffing, they were overworked every day. I saw care aides that could bathe and dress a patient at super speed. It was efficient, but not gentle. It isn't that the staff didn't care. Rather, there just wasn't time to give each patient the attention they deserved. When you have to get multiple patients up, time is at a premium and care suffers.

Going back to my first patient, I remember arriving one morning to find him feeling ill and freezing cold. It turned out that his bedside window had been open all night, and so he had not gotten any sleep. He had tried to ring for help, but his call bell had been broken for months, and no one had been able to fix it yet. Events like this were common, and it has since gotten worse rather than better.

. . .

Second year is a bit of a blur to me, so many years later. There will probably be some third-year stuff mixed in here as well. If I get a few of the details wrong, I hope that you will forgive me. I am sure that my fellow students will gladly point out any mistakes that I have made.

Our second year began with a special event for the nursing students. Back in our first year, I had signed up to be a student representative for our professional organization. Each year of the program had two representatives, and we met together about once a month to discuss various issues. One of the needs that my co-representative and I had identified in our first year was the need for more mentors. The nursing students in other years were always so busy that we barely had any contact with them. Even when we did, they always seemed rather unapproachable. Because of this, the students in all four years had become very disconnected from one another. As lowly first years, many of us felt that we could not approach those further along in the program for guidance when we needed it.

Once we, as student representatives, had identified this need, we knew that something had to be done about it. Together, we decided that the best way to combat this feeling of being isolated was to organize a day when all the nursing students got together. We got food and organized games and other activities for everyone. The instructors liked the idea so much, they decreed that all nursing students had to attend, no excuses. Once again, my sense of irony kicked in. Because everyone *had* to go, I dubbed the event "mandatory fun day" and the name stuck. I'm not sure if they still do it, but I know that it became a tradition for several years afterwards. I do remember my ex-wife once wondering aloud who had come up with such a stupid idea. I can't recall if I admitted to my crime. Probably not.

As for our classes, I vividly remember taking pathobiology. For those of you that don't know, pathobiology is the study of diseases and disease processes. The first semester I enjoyed immensely because it was all about how diseases progress. This appealed to my inquisitive brain, as I'm sure you can imagine. Again, we explored how all disease processes interconnect and how they can affect multiple systems. More of those three-dimensional puzzles to figure out. The course was also taught by the same instructor that had taught our anatomy course, so it was again very nursing focused. I learned a great deal.

Our second semester of pathobiology was a whole other story. We had a new instructor, so it wasn't quite as focused. The course was all about bacteria and infection, and it involved a great deal of memorization. I should tell you that whatever part of the brain is responsible for remembering names has never functioned very well for me. In fact, I have always struggled to remember names. I even go out of my way to avoid introducing people because I am always afraid that I will forget one of their names. I think that some of my friends have always thought me a bit rude because of this. They always glance at me with a confused look in their eyes, before giving up and introducing themselves. Now they know why I do it. My dirty little secret is out.

As a result of my poor memorization skills, trying to remember the names of all the different types of bacteria and what kind of infections they caused proved very difficult for me. I had no idea what I was doing most of the time. I believe I passed the second semester by a single question on the final exam. We needed 60 percent to pass, and I ended up with a grade of 60.01 percent. Hardly my finest hour.

...

At some point during second year, I heard that people from the other programs were complaining about the nursing students. They thought we were snobby because we would always eat lunch as a group, rather than mingling. People actually thought we harbored the belief that we were better than everyone else. I thought, "Who the hell would want to eat lunch with us?" Our conversations were not exactly stimulating for the appetite most of the time, if you get my meaning.

By far, the best part of second year was clinical. That year, we started in the very first semester, and we were in the hospital proper. My group began on the medical floor. Others began on the surgical floor, and we switched around for second semester. I absolutely loved it, mainly because it was all very task oriented. It was exciting and dynamic, and we finally got to do stuff. Of course, we were still closely supervised at first. Once we had successfully demonstrated a skill (such as inserting a catheter), however, we were allowed to do it on our own from that point on. I remember that many of us carried little lists in our pockets of the skills we still needed to demonstrate, and we would check them off as we completed each one. We had our own patients to look after, but if a procedure came up for another patient, we were encouraged to jump in and do it. I was always one of the first to volunteer.

I also noticed that many of my fellow students had started coming to me for advice. I was never a great classroom student, but I really came out of my shell in clinical, and I was good at it. There is a saying amongst nurses that goes, "Fake it till you make it." It means that we should exude confidence, even when we aren't confident at all. I guess that I was simply better at acting. Everyone seemed to think that I knew what I was doing, even though I certainly didn't feel that way at the time.

Our instructor was fantastic. She was an ER nurse, and she had the wickedest sense of humor. At least I thought so; it would probably be a little too dark for most people. Some of the other students found her a little intimidating. She pushed us hard during clinical, but in an encouraging way. Most of us were wallflowers at the beginning of the semester, but she wasn't having any of it. If the opportunity to perform a new procedure came up, she would quickly come grab one of us and shove us in there. By doing this, we were able to experience much more than we would have if left to our own devices. More than that, we began to see that many aspects of nursing care were nowhere near as difficult as we might have imagined. Each success built on the ones before, so she really helped each of us to grow and to find our confidence. I don't think that any of us would have seen half as much if not for her. She was my favorite instructor during the nursing program.

I believe it was also in second year that I had to spend a week on maternity (we all did). There is nothing quite as sad as a male nursing student on maternity because we don't get to do a whole lot. This is perfectly understandable. Many expectant mothers did not relish the idea of having some strange man in the room while they were giving birth. As a result, I spent most of my time hanging IV medications. I did get to see a Cesarean section, which was amazing. I also managed to get in on one delivery, and I'm pretty sure that it was on the very last day we were there. Luckily, she was already pretty far into labor when we arrived on the ward. Because of how far along she was, I am sure that Elvis and a herd of dancing unicorns could have asked to come in and she wouldn't have cared. After it was all over, the maternity nurse had the placenta inside a metal bowl. She held it up so that we could all see. I am not ashamed to admit that this was the only time in my entire nursing career where I have felt queasy. I thought that I was seriously going to throw up.

During our second semester, we were on the surgical floor. Again, we spent a great deal of time just trying to find skills to practice. There was a lot of wound care. It was very similar to first semester, so I don't really recall anything in particular. To be quite honest, I have never been that interested in caring for surgical patients anyway.

One event from our surgical rotation stands out for me, however. At some point, I got to spend a day in the OR. This was a smaller hospital, so we didn't do open heart surgery or anything like that. What we did a lot of was orthopedic surgeries, such as hip replacements. Now, if any of my readers are going in for orthopedic surgery soon, you might want to skip over this next bit.

As a guy, watching an orthopedic surgery is really the coolest thing ever. There are all these huge tools that the surgeons use, so it's like being on the set of *Home Improvement*. I'm not even kidding. They look very similar to the tools you would find at any hardware store, only a whole lot bigger. Once the patient is sedated and the appropriate incision is made, the surgeon grabs one of these tools and goes to work. Suddenly, the room is filled with this great cacophony of grinding and whirring. You can see smoke and bone dust rising up out of the wound. Had I not become a nurse, I think that orthopedic surgeon would have topped my list of career choices.

The nurses who work in the OR are also quite skilled. They are like ninja nurses. I swear to you, an OR nurse can pass between two sterile fields three inches apart without bumping either one. I could never do what they do. I am a terrible klutz, and I know that I would be knocking things over every time I turned around. I would have gotten fired as a surgical nurse very quickly.

Despite my fascination with the surgery itself, I was really there to observe what the nurses did. At some point, one of the nurses told me that I would be able to see the surgery better if I moved to a certain spot. They were quite surprised when I told them that I was not there to see the surgeon work. I was there to see the nurses work. I wanted to know what they did. As nurses, we so often sell ourselves short, I think. We are not less than doctors, we are different, and we both have very important roles to play. Without surgical nurses, there would be no surgeries at all.

There was one other event that had a great impact on me. I was looking after a palliative patient who simply refused to die. He was clinging to life with a stubbornness that puzzled us greatly. On one occasion, I entered the room and found his wife sitting at the bedside. Her face looked as if it had been carved from stone, as if she was trying desperately to hold her emotions in check. I busied myself with the patient for a few minutes, and then I turned my attention to her. I asked her if she needed anything. Suddenly, she broke down and cried. In between sobs, she told me that in all the times she had visited her husband, not once had anyone given her any attention. I was the first.

We ended up talking for quite a while. During our conversation, I realized how scared was about losing her husband. Not only was she sad at the prospect of losing him, but she also felt a profound sense of helplessness. Apparently, during their many years together, he had managed most of the finances and other such details. She had no idea where to even begin without him, which served to amplify her fear. I was able to offer understanding that helped ease her fears. Feeling more confident in her own abilities, she was able to say goodbye to her husband at last. He died a few hours later, and to this day I am certain that it was his concern for his wife that had kept him going for so long. Once he felt that she was going to be ok, he was able to let go.

. . .

We also had several goodbyes that year. Apparently, second year is the weeding out year in nursing school, so many of our fellow students were asked to leave. I think we lost about a quarter of our class. Nursing school is a rather intense experience. It is filled with sleepless nights, endless assignments, and way too much coffee and alcohol. An environment like that breeds a certain closeness, so every single loss hit us very deeply. It was somewhat like having a limb severed, as if a big part of us had suddenly gone missing. It also instilled in us a great deal of fear and paranoia, as we were each left to wonder if we would be next.

. . .

Third year was the year of electives. We had to do three electives in total, with the first one having been completed already. There was quite a wide range of choices, depending on what our interests were. However, whatever we chose had to be somehow related to nursing.

Many of us chose to take a pharmacology course, just because it was offered right at the college. That is weeks of my life I will never get back. They had an actual pharmacist come in to teach the class, so I am quite sure that there was a ton of useful information provided to us. Unfortunately, the instructor was quite possibly the most boring person ever to walk the earth. To make matters worse, she possessed one of those monotone voices that puts everyone to sleep. Because of this, I don't think any of us absorbed a single thing. It was often a struggle just to remain awake.

For the second elective, most of the choices we were given were correspondence courses. Now, you will recall that I had a pretty clear idea of where I wanted to work, even before attending nursing school. Therefore, I chose to begin my ER specialty course that year. This program was offered at a nearby university and consisted of three academic courses and two clinicals. We only needed to complete one credit, but, for some strange reason, the first academic course did not count. It had to be the second academic course. As a result, I had two courses to get through instead of just one. A few of my fellow students were in the same boat, but most avoided the specialty courses for this very reason. They signed up for simpler courses instead.

It was most definitely not an easy course either. Specialty courses are very focused, and there is a great deal of technical knowledge that the student must absorb. There is also an assumption that the student is already an RN, so they build on concepts that the student should have already mastered while in nursing school. As a direct result, much of the foundational information was simply not covered. I, however, was still learning a lot of the basics. In order to keep up, I was forced to learn things that we had not yet covered in school.

Trying to juggle nursing school and an advanced elective was exhausting. Many times, I really wished that I had chosen something easier. I could have done the ER course after nursing school instead and had a much easier time of it. I did manage to get through the first course, mostly because my instructor was very patient with me. The second course was much harder, and this time I had to drop out. The reality is that I was not even close to meeting the deadlines for my assignments. In all, I think I started the course three times before I was able to get all the way through to the end. In fact, it took so long that I very nearly ran out of time. In order to graduate, we had to submit all our final grades by a certain date. I believe that my final grade for the ER course was received on the very last day.

Third year was also the year of community health, which covers both home care and public health. During the first semester, we spent time doing both.

For those not familiar, home care involves caring for people in their own homes. Some of the patients had post-op incisions that needed to be looked after. Others were immobile and so required care for pressure ulcers. There was a wide variety of other reasons people required home care, as well.

I got a real surprise while I was in home care. I found that I absolutely loved it. Beforehand, I had not thought that I would. After all, it seemed very far removed from my chosen field in emergency. The two do have striking similarities, however. There is a great deal of autonomy, and the nurses must be able to think on their feet. In home care, the nurses are out on their own seeing clients (they are never referred to as patients in home care), so being comfortable with independence is a must. Also, they are never able to predict how the day will play out. That unknown quality is another aspect that the two have in common.

I found wound care fascinating. There were a thousand different types of dressings, and they all had very specific purposes. Some of them promote new tissue growth, some kill off bacteria, while some help get rid of dead tissue. Knowing what each type of dressing did was essential. To be honest, I learned more about wound care in that one semester than I have throughout the rest of my career. When I eventually began working in the ER, I often had opportunities to pass that knowledge along.

It is also a very different experience looking after people in their homes. For starters, I was now on their turf. With a few exceptions (no guns, no loose dogs, etc.) it's essentially "their house, their rules." That is very different from the hospital setting. Often, the clients would sit and watch TV or read while we worked. They also often knew more about their own wound care than the nurses did. Many were very specific about their care, right down to what dressings we were supposed to be using.

Another aspect of being on their turf was that sometimes we had to get very creative. I remember once being in a woman's home and she needed to have a urinary catheter inserted. Now, to make the situation even more complex, this was to be my first female catheterization. The problem was that the patient was completely immobile. Also, her bed was right up against the wall, so there was no room to properly position myself for the procedure. I ended up having to climb onto the bed, and then I had to straddle her. So, there I am: I had my knees on either side of her pelvis, I had my head between her knees, and I had to feed this catheter in upside down. Female catheters were never really a challenge for me again. In fact, by comparison, they all seemed to be rather simple.

As students, we were also able to advocate for changes. Nurses often tend to believe that we know better than the students. However, those students are often able to provide updated information that we may not be aware of. After all, they have access to the latest available research. Often, they also have recently practiced skills that we have long forgotten, just because they are skills that we rarely use. Many times, throughout my career, I have relied on students to teach me on certain subjects. While we were students in home care, we had one such opportunity. As it turned out, the home care nurses had recently switched from latex gloves to vinyl, both to cut costs and to avoid latex allergies. Much to their surprise, we informed them that vinyl gloves should never be used in a medical setting because they don't actually protect from any blood or bodily fluids. They are too porous. There was quite the uproar after we revealed that little tidbit of information. I was even able to provide several studies in support of this, and soon home care had switched to nitryl gloves (the blue ones). These provide the protection of latex without the hazards, though they cost a great deal more.

By contrast, public health was not my favorite placement. I remember a lot of sitting, which did not suit me. I believe that my bum actually started to go numb. By the end of our placement, I seriously thought that I was going to need an ass transplant. It's not that public health nurses don't work hard, don't get me wrong. It's just a different kind of work. It's a lot more like an office job. A great deal of research, phone calls, that sort of thing. It just wasn't my cup of tea. I found it a little too dry.

I also remember having a few concerns while I was there. Public health often does home visits for newborns. This is just to check in and see how things are going, especially with first-time moms. On one such visit, the baby's grandmother was also present, and she turned out to be a former nurse herself. Because of the grandmother's presence, the public health nurse proceeded to bypass the mother entirely. All her questions were directed to the grandmother instead. Now, I can understand perfectly why this occurred. It is always much easier to talk with someone who knows the lingo, after all. Still, the mother was obviously feeling excluded, especially as we had come to check up on her. I believe that I asked the nurse about it later, but she didn't really have an answer for me. To tell the truth, I am not even sure that she had been aware of what she was doing.

Another concerning incident happened when I was present at an immunization clinic. It had been specifically set up for people with schizophrenia. Now, for legal purposes, there has to be consent from the patient before we can give them a shot. To speed the process along, nurses will often assume that if you are lining up to get a shot, you are also consenting to the shot. In this case, however, I felt like that wasn't sufficient. I suspected that a few of the patients didn't really understand what was going on. When I asked one gentleman why he was lining up, he told me it was because everyone else was. Nobody had really discussed the immunizations with the patients beforehand. Because of this, I did not feel that we had met the legal and ethical standards for informed consent.

I was so disturbed by these occurrences that I even talked to my instructor about them. She made me "reflect" on each incident in my journal. She then insisted that I rewrite my reflections three times. She didn't feel that I was getting the wording right, despite the fact that I obviously understood the concepts because we had discussed them at length. I felt the writing to be a bit redundant, never mind having to write it out more than once.

...

During third year, we were given a choice about where to go for our last practicums. I had enjoyed home care so much that I chose to return. This was also the first time we were doing practicums with a preceptor guiding us, rather than one of our instructors. Preceptors are nurses who work in a given area and have agreed to take on students. We would follow the same preceptor around for however long we remained in our chosen area. I think that this was the first time I had ever felt like an actual nurse. My preceptor always talked to me as a colleague, rather than as a student. We would discuss different aspects of care, and I always felt that my opinion was heard and valued. By the end of the semester, I was even doing some of the care myself.

The only drawback was that home care had eight-hour shifts, instead of twelve-hour shifts like in the hospital. It took me about two weeks longer to get my required hours done, so most of my fellow students were already on vacation before I was.

...

Just before our summer break in third year, we received some incredible news. The government had devised a plan that would allow us to work as student nurses, as long as we did not try to exceed our current level of training. We were the first class of nursing students to be granted this privilege. Of course, we were all very excited about this opportunity. For the first time, we were going to experience what it was like to work as real nurses. More than that, we would be getting paid for our work. We weren't on our own or anything even remotely like that. Instead, we would work with the regular nurses, but we would have tasks of our own to complete. This provided us with a real sense of responsibility for our own practice. It also provided us with some much-needed cash. I was able to quit my regular job as a result. Finally, no more minimum wage.

I ended up taking a position in pediatrics. I really enjoy working with children and even considered pursuing a career in emergency pediatric nursing for a while. Unfortunately, though it was a great learning experience, it wasn't quite what I had been hoping for. Besides, the nurse manager really didn't seem to like me much. I had originally wanted to apply to the ER, but I figured that they would not be taking any student nurses. As it turned out, I was wrong. One of my classmates applied for and got a position there. I started to drop by whenever things were slow in pediatrics, and before long I had finagled a position there instead. The manager in pediatrics didn't even try to talk me out of leaving.

That was such an incredible experience. I had never worked in an ER before, so I had no idea what to expect, of course. It was nothing like on TV, that was for sure. It was always a lot busier, for starters. I have noticed that ERs on TV never seem to have many patients. Despite being so busy, the experience did cement my desire to work in the ER, once I was officially qualified. While I was there, I always saw it as my role to make the nurses' lives easier, in any way I could. I helped with patients, and I also did a lot of the stocking up for the department. I learned how to put patients on the monitors, what the more common heart rhythms looked like (you would be amazed to discover just how many there actually are), how to properly assess patients, and how to treat various injuries. In other words, I was having the time of my life.

There were also events that exposed me to some of the flaws in the system. This was a smaller hospital, and a rather underfunded one at that. At night, there was often only one ER nurse. There was also a critical care float, who helped out in both the ER and the ICU. If they really got stuck, the hospital's head nurse would also come and help. On many shifts, they also had me or the other student. Still, that is not a whole lot of people. Most of the time, it all worked out ok. Still, there were a few times that I was in way over my head, simply because there was nobody else around. I remember once being the only nurse available for a trauma that had just arrived. I kept sticking my head out of the door and calling for help, hoping that someone was going to come to my rescue. To be clear, it wasn't that I didn't know what to do. I simply wasn't qualified or licensed to be in there on my own. I was only a student, after all. Somebody did come in after about ten minutes, but I had to basically drag them into the trauma room. At the time, it felt like a great deal longer than ten minutes.

...

Fourth year came at last. There's something peculiar that happens to a person's psyche when they get close to a goal, or to the end of a long journey. Anyone who's ever ridden a horse will tell you that you have to hold the reigns just a little bit tighter when you are heading back to the barn. The same was true for us nursing students.

By fourth year, we were all extremely tired and more than a little fed up. For three years, we had not had any sleep. We had also not seen a lot of our friends and family. It had taken a definite toll on us. I can remember the mood being just a little tense that year. Not amongst ourselves, mind you, because we never turned on each other. We were quite ready, however, to take on anyone else unlucky enough to cross our paths. We had started to resemble a pack of wild dogs, ready to attack anyone who threatened the pack. Also, we all looked a little shaggy, hungry, and rabid by this point. This was probably due to the lack of sleep, I suspect.

I specifically remember one day, toward the end of the first semester. We were upset about one of our final assignments because it was taking forever to mark for some reason. In frustration, we all went out to lunch that day. I imagine that we lost track of time because we arrived back late for classes. Needless to say, the instructors were not pleased with us, and they told us so. Their admonishment hit a raw nerve and all our irritation just came pouring out. We told them that they represented none of the values that they were trying to instill in us. Harsh, I know. I do feel bad about this episode, but I think that this is as close to an apology as I am ever going to make on the matter.

Somehow, we did manage to get through that first semester without killing or seriously maiming anyone. Still, I imagine that we were not at all pleasant to be around. Luckily, as we did not have clinical placements, all our time was spent in the classroom. No one else had to experience the foulness of our collective tempers. That was our last academic semester, which is why we were so eager to just have it over and done with.

The second and third semesters were all clinical. I think I must have done a little happy dance the last day of actual classes. I'm sure we all did. It was just such a relief to finally be done.

For my winter practicum, I had chosen, wait for it...emergency. Shocker, right? I had chosen three excellent preceptors to work with. I needed three was because all of them worked only part-time. One of them was also on vacation for part of my practicum. It took all of them combined to make up the full-time hours I would need. It was not, as some of you might be thinking, because they could only stand to be around me for short periods of time.

My first preceptor was one of the smartest nurses I have ever worked with. She was also one of the most professional. I don't think I ever saw anything get her worked up. She was full of boundless energy and always wore a smile. Also, she was very "by the book," and this provided me with a solid foundation for my own practice.

The second was also very smart, and she questioned me mercilessly. I mean that in a good way. She pushed me to really think about what I was doing and why I was doing it, rather than to just do tasks. I really had to be able to justify my choices whenever I was working with her. This inspired me to always dig deeper because understanding means that we give better care and make fewer mistakes. Because of my time with her, I have striven to make understanding the cornerstone of my entire nursing practice. Now, whenever I have had students of my own, I do the exact same thing with them. I am sure that a few of my former students are rolling their eyes as they read these words. Now they all know whom to blame.

My third preceptor was just about the nicest ER nurse I have ever met. She was always patient with me, and she always took the time to explain things. She was also fairly new to the ER, so she understood some of what I was going through. I felt less intimidated whenever I worked with her. She helped me to develop a greater sense of confidence in myself.

They are three incredible women, and I cannot praise them enough.

One lesson I learned during that time was how little I actually knew. Nothing that I had learned in school had prepared me for the real thing. One of the complaints I often hear about new nurses (I hear a lot of complaints, but most of them are not even worth putting down on paper) is that they don't know what they don't know. That lesson was driven home for me over and over again during my practicum, sometimes even painfully. I had assumed that working there as a student nurse would better prepare me for the environment. I was very, very wrong. Now, I was expected to know stuff. I wasn't just stocking up and helping out where I could anymore. At least I already knew my way around the place, so I was never stuck looking for things. I had managed to pick up *some* knowledge along the way, after all, so I wasn't exactly starting from scratch. In addition, I also had the first two ER courses under my belt, which provided me with a great foundation to build upon. Still, it was a very different environment to the one I had gotten used to. There was now a level of responsibility that had been absent up until this point. There is also a huge difference between knowing facts, and seeing those facts put into action. I do think that I succeeded, just not very gracefully. There were a lot of bumps along the way.

For my third and final semester, I went back to the medical floor. At that time, no one ever went straight from nursing school into a specialty area, such as the ER. It was expected that new nurses gain experience first. I was sure that I was going to have to do floor nursing for a few years before I could get a position down in the emergency room, or before I even thought of applying. That is why I decided to do my final practicum on a medical ward. I really needed the experience, and I wanted that experience to be fresh after I graduated. At this point, I had not done any floor nursing since my second year, so I really needed the refresher.

For this practicum, I only had one preceptor.

I can still remember my first day being there. The first task that nurses do when they start a shift is to check on all the patients they have been assigned. Like a good nurse, I went off to do just that. When I returned to my preceptor about half an hour later, she appeared quite surprised to see me so soon. I think she assumed that, since I had returned so quickly, I hadn't done a very good job of it. This is where I think my emergency experience really paid off. I was able to tell her everything I had done and everything that I had seen in detail. I was used to being quick and efficient with my assessments, so I had just gone at it.

Of course, I was still very inexperienced. As a result, I did make several silly mistakes. One of my first days up there, I was looking after a patient and I dropped a sterile object that he needed on the floor. I had foolishly untied it when I should not have done so. To be clear, there is absolutely no five-second rule in the hospital. Anything that lands on our floors usually ends up in the garbage. However, we did not have a replacement in this case, so tossing it was simply not an option. I quickly grabbed the object and stuck it in a glass filled with sterile water. I let it soak first, then I scrubbed it vigorously to clean it. Once it had been thoroughly sanitized, I gently placed it back where it belonged. Crisis averted. Still, I was absolutely mortified. My preceptor had been off doing something else at the time. When she returned, I confessed my error. Instead of reprimanding me, she seemed genuinely impressed. At least, she told me she was. In reality, she might have just been trying to placate the dumb guy. I had made an error, for sure. However, I had remained calm, I had fixed the problem, and I had admitted to it. Now, I am not telling this tale to brag. Well, not *just* to brag anyway. It was another big learning moment for me. I strongly believe that, as nurses, we have to be accountable above all else. To this day, I am still the first one to say something when I make a mistake.

As I mentioned earlier, the one aspect of being a student that I sorely miss is being able to spend more quality time with my patients. In those days, I wasn't so consumed by everything that needed to get done. During my practicum, there was an incident that has always stayed with me. It was the first shift that I was going to take the entire team. In other words, I was supposed to do everything that night. Instead, I went into my first patient's room, and everything went horribly wrong. We were chatting away, when she suddenly passed out and went very pale. I was in an absolute panic, of course. Despite my experience in the ER, I believe that this was my first true code blue situation. Fortunately, my ER training took over once again. I was just about to scream for help (and I do mean scream), but in that moment my brain kicked in. I knew that she had a do-not-resuscitate order and that we were not going to do anything to fix her condition anyway. Ok, deep breath. Once I had calmed down, I stuck my head out the door and called for my preceptor. I explained the situation to her and asked if she could take the rest of the team to start out, which she agreed to do. I then went back into the room, sat by the patient's bedside, and just held her hand until she died about half an hour later. I was so thankful that she didn't have to die alone. I truly miss being able to do things like that. However, when you are a nurse, there is no one to take over for you as my preceptor did. You are it, and the other patients need you as well. If I had been an actual nurse at that time, I would have been forced to move on.

This brings to mind another story. I found this event a little funny, but then I possess a very twisted sense of humor, which is the same for all nurses, ever!. I think it was on one of our first nights together, and we had just started our shift. My preceptor and I entered one of the rooms and found an elderly woman reading aloud to one of the patients. She looked up when we entered and informed us that her friend was taking a nap because she hadn't been feeling very well earlier. You can see where this is going, right? One look at the patient and we knew that, not only was she dead, but she was quite thoroughly dead. Probably had been for a few hours at least. All the while, her friend had been patiently reading to her.

Speaking of dead people, it was during this practicum that I had to take a body down to the morgue for the very first time. Yes, it is exactly as creepy as it sounds. When we got down there, we had to take the body from the cart and place it on a table that is used for performing autopsies. We were moving the body over when I dropped the head. It didn't hit the table hard, but there was still a loud, hollow thud. I think my heart stopped, right there. I had to keep repeating to myself, "It didn't hurt him, it didn't hurt him." I was justifiably horrified.

There was another patient that I would like to talk about because he also had a big impact on my practice. He was a gentleman who had fallen from his bike with no helmet on. For the rest of his days, he was unable to perform even the simplest of tasks for himself. Because of this, I have become an unwavering advocate for wearing helmets. If you had presented to the ER after wiping out on your bike, you had better have been wearing one. If not, there was a very stern lecture coming. Many kids where I live do not seem to wear helmets, for some reason. They seem to think that it is death-defying. I am here to tell you death is not the worst thing that can happen to a person. Wear your helmet!

Just like the ER, the floors experience the same issues, but in their own way. The floor I was on was supposed to house medical patients. Instead, half of the patients on most days were waiting for placement in care homes. We call these patients ALC (alternative level of care). They represent one of the biggest challenges in health care today. They need care, but they don't really need *hospital* care. There are so few spaces in care homes, that they can often end up languishing for months while waiting for a spot to open up.

I remember during my final practicum that one of these ALC patients used to stand next to the elevator doors. He would greet people as they came to visit their loved ones. He had dementia and would occasionally do this stark naked. It was a bit of a shock for some of the visitors as they stepped from the elevator.

I just want to give you an idea of how large this problem is. Right now, in the hospital where I currently work, there are over sixty of these ALC patients. That is sixty beds that we are unable to use for acute patients who are being admitted. The patients who actually need hospital care. Those sixty beds represent 16 percent of our total bed space. That is a travesty.

...

And then, I was done. The four years of hell were now over. I had somehow managed to get all my ducks in a row, and I had even managed to pass everything. I am sure that a few of my instructors were surprised by this, but no one was more surprised than me. There was a bit of a rush at the end, trying to get my final grade for the ER course in. However, after a day spent making several frantic phone calls, even that fell into place at the last possible moment.

This is when the other shoe dropped. Back before we even started nursing school, we all had to have a criminal record check done. This, of course, makes sense. It's a way to protect patients, particularly children. The problem was that I actually had a criminal record. It was all very minor offences, and nothing violent. I had informed our professional organization of this before even starting the program, and once they had received a copy of my actual record, they were just fine with it.

Flash forward four years to graduation time. Our professional organization had gone through some major changes while we were in fourth year. Even the name was different. After I had slogged through four years of nursing school, they suddenly decided that they were no longer ok with my record. I received a very nicely worded letter, informing me that they would not be issuing me a license to practice after all. I was both devastated and incredibly angry. Just as I was about to cross the finish line, they had completely changed the rules on me. Four years of my life had been totally wasted, not to mention the thousands of dollars in debt I had just accumulated.

I begged, I pleaded. My case went back and forth between this committee and that, with each one standing firm on their decision. By now, I was absolutely livid. I wrote them a very *nicely* worded letter outlining exactly where they could stick their license. Luckily, one of my instructors read my letter and talked me out of sending it. Instead, I sent a very heartfelt letter, telling them what a great asset I would be to the nursing profession. I included recommendations from many of my preceptors and instructors. I reminded them that I had even spent four years as a student representative for their organization. Whatever I said, it worked. They relented and gave me my license to practice. Big sigh of relief there.

Now, it was officially time to celebrate. As nursing students, we have two graduation ceremonies. First, we have the official graduation. This took place in a large gymnasium, and the graduates from each program at the college were present. We had to wear gowns and everything. Everyone's families were also in attendance, and the room was very crowded. It was very warm, especially with our gowns on. I am surprised that none of us passed out. One by one, we were called up to the podium to receive our degrees. There was a photographer present, but for some odd reason he only seemed to take shots of the backs of our heads. We were then expected to buy these pictures as mementoes. Luckily, my mother had managed to get some good photos of me.

The second ceremony was our pinning. This was just for the nursing students and our families. This ceremony is done to mark the transition from nursing student to nurse, and each of us receives a pin with the school logo on it. It is considered a rite of passage for all nurses, and all nursing schools hold similar ceremonies.

At this point, many of you are probably thinking that we were finished at last. School was now behind us. That is not how it works, however. You see, once we have graduated from the nursing program, we become full-fledged nurses. To work, though, we need to be *registered* nurses. That means we must also pass the dreaded nursing exam. Let me fill you in on the details.

To start, this is an all-day exam administered by our professional organization. When I took it, there were two separate parts to the exam. In the morning, it was multiple choice questions on a wide variety of nursing subjects. In fact, there seemed to be an inordinate amount of questions on maternity and public health, neither of which are among my strongest areas of expertise.

In the afternoon, we had short answers. They are tricky too. One of the strategies you learn quickly as a student is how to obfuscate. In a written exam, this is where you are not sure of the answer, so you just ramble on endlessly in the hopes that the correct answer is in there somewhere. In the nursing exam, you can't do this. They give you a dotted line, and you are not allowed to write anything more than what will fit on that line. How cruel is that?

Apparently, the next year, they were forced to do away with the written portion of the exam. Someone had leaked the answers online, so they canceled the second half of the exam and just never brought it back again. Lucky bastards.

When the day of the exam came, there were a few hundred of us. They used a central location, so a few different schools were represented. We were all brought into a large gymnasium, where they proceeded to administer a security check on us that would put the Secret Service to shame. We were allowed one pencil and one pencil sharpener. That was it. Water was provided for us, just in case anyone had tried to smuggle answers in by stuffing them inside of a bottle. If we needed to go to the bathroom, we were escorted.

I want to say something important to any nursing students that might be reading this. They have since changed the exam again, but what I am going to say still holds true. You will come out of that room feeling like you failed. That is normal. Every single one of you will feel that way. You probably didn't. That is all.

Of course, I did pass the exam. One of the curious things is that they never tell us how we did. It's only you passed or you failed. I have no idea how well I did or what my score was. Still, it was finally done. I was now officially an RN.

GET A JOB
(SHA NA NA NA, SHA NA NA NA NA)

To begin, I would like to apologize for the title of this chapter. I am sure many of you will now be singing that song in your head for the rest of the day. The crueler part of me finds that extraordinarily funny.

If you have no idea what I am talking about, you are far too young to be a nurse!

After graduation, my first thought was, "Now what happens?" Let me tell you, being a student nurse and being an actual nurse are two very different things. For starters, as a student you might be looking after patients of your own, but the ultimate responsibility is always someone else's. As a nurse, suddenly they are *your* patients. That is a very different distinction. That transition can be very unsettling, to say the least.

There is a strange thing that happens once you start life as a real nurse. Four years of education completely vanishes from your mind, like a puff of smoke. Suddenly, you don't remember a damn thing. It's as if there has been a complete brain wipe of all that accumulated knowledge. As a student, I had always felt fairly confident. On my first job, I felt like the stupidest person alive. I didn't seem to know anything anymore, so I blundered around just hoping that no one would notice. It is a very uncomfortable feeling, and it takes about two full years to dissipate completely.

Also, as a student, no one really cares what you do or when. There is simply the expectation that it will all get done. As a nurse, suddenly you're on a schedule, and you can't just toddle of for break whenever you feel like it. You are part of a team now, and you need to go on break when they tell you to go on break. If you don't, everyone else will hate you because all their breaks are now delayed as well.

I had managed to secure a position in the ER, but as a medical nurse. It was in the same local hospital where I had done all my training. My job was to care for the admitted patients. I also continued to help the ER nurses where I could, but that was unofficial and not part of my assigned duties. There was a room down the hall that often housed admitted patients, and there were often admitted patients scattered about in the halls as well.

The government had developed another big program for new graduates. The government agreed to pay our wages for a full year so that our pay did not come out of the hospital budgets. This was meant to provide an incentive to hire us because we were essentially free labor for the hospitals. I believe that my new position had been specifically created just for me. This would never have been possible without the new program.

During those first days, my biggest stressor was believing that I had to complete every task before the end of my shift. At the end of my day, I would often be left scrambling, trying to get those last few items completed before the next shift arrived. This is another curious thing about new nurses (though I know plenty of more experienced nurses who do this as well): that mindset that we must hand over a clean slate at the end of every shift. There is also the mindset that we should always have a clean slate handed to us at the beginning of each shift. As I have matured in my practice, I have realized that this is not always possible or necessary. No one should be standing around all day, and no one should be passing off *all* their work to others. If you are busy, however, there is no shame in not completing every little thing. This is why hospitals are open twenty-four hours a day. There is always another shift after you.

I also learned the value of asking questions. For some reason, this was a big fear of mine at the beginning. It all goes back to that fear of appearing stupid. As a result, I made an error that I have not been able to let go of in all the years since. It was during one of my first shifts, and I was looking after three patients. I had been told that, as a medical nurse, I was not to touch the monitors in any way. During the night, I was not sure how vitals were to be recorded (taking vitals is part of what the monitors do). I'm also not sure why the patients were on the monitors to begin with, as they were admitted patients. Anyway, the point is that I was afraid to ask, so I just left it. Instead, I had simply assumed that someone else would be recording them. As a result, no vital signs had been written down throughout the entire shift. I received quite the reprimand the next day.

One of the things that made those first few months bearable was knowing that I was not alone. One of my closest friends and classmates worked on the maternity ward, and our schedules often overlapped. This meant that we were often able to spend our breaks together, which afforded us the opportunity to compare notes. There is something very soothing in knowing that others are suffering just as you are. There were also other classmates who worked around the hospital, and sometimes I would hang out with them during breaks. I am very thankful that we were able to support one another during those first days as new grads.

Perhaps one of the most unnerving aspects of the job was looking after admitted psychiatric patients. It didn't happen very often, thankfully. In fact, I think it only happened twice while I was there. One of the things we do very badly in emergency rooms is look after psych patients. This is not because we are mean or cruel. It is simply the nature of the environment. When looking after people who are injured or critically ill, we can never afford to be distracted. Therefore, all *potential* distractions need to be contained. For psych patients, we literally had a cell with a locked door. In this room they would remain, until the psychiatric department could take them. I have seen patients languish in these rooms for days on end, while they wait for an inpatient bed to become available. Needless to say, the patients do not take kindly to this. Being locked up can increases their agitation and makes their behavior even more unpredictable. Often, we had to enter the room to give medications and do assessments. This could be a very volatile situation, and it was a task I did not ever look forward to.

There was one more lesson that I learned very quickly. It is something that all new nurses discover. It is to "beware the unexplained wet spot." I am sure that needs no explanation.

I believe I mentioned at one point about how tight funds were at this hospital. That is mostly because this was one of the few remaining private hospitals around, and the way that they kept this cozy little arrangement going was to keep costs as low as possible. As a result, our hospital operated at approximately 70 percent of the budget of a similar sized hospital else-where. Of course, the only way to achieve this was to cut as many corners as possible. There was never enough staff, the hospital was in serious need of upgrades, and the atmosphere was dark and oppressive. I would comment on how this affected staff morale, but there really was no staff morale to speak of. Every single person there seemed upset most of the time. Stress leave was common, as you can imagine. I do not remember ever feeling welcomed or valued by those in positions of authority.

In the medical field, there are institutions known as magnet hospitals. These are hospitals that attract staff because they make the well-being of staff a priority. This was not our hospital. I remember commenting to one of the doctors that we probably qualified as a *repellent* hospital instead. He actually used my statement in a board meeting once, trying to describe the environment to management. Didn't seem to help at all.

My close friend, the one I would hang out with all the time, left her job a few years after I did. Her stress level was so high that she has been unable to work as a nurse since.

· · ·

At some point (I believe that it was about six months after I had started), the rules determining who could take the emergency nursing course were changed. To recruit more specialty nurses, the course was now available free of charge. Previously, I would have had to pay for it myself. In addition, they were no longer requiring two years of floor experience beforehand, and the length of the course had been condensed. Finally, it was also decided that nurses would continue to earn a paycheck while taking the course. I must admit, I was a little surprised when our manager put my name forward as a candidate. Still, I was pretty excited about the whole thing. It was a great opportunity.

I got off to a very bad start. That is because I missed my first two class sessions. See, the classroom portion was quite far away, about a three-hour drive. Because of this, I had to get up very early both days for the trip. Well, that first day I got about halfway there and one of my front tires blew out. Luckily, I was passing through a large town, and so I managed to get the tire changed without too much difficulty. By that time, though, I had pretty much missed the day, so I returned home. I repeated the process the next morning, and damned if my other front tire didn't blow out. This time, it decided to blow near the same town, but quite a bit further down the highway.

Oh, and by the way, I had gotten my driver's license by this point. A friend insisted I put this in here, in case some of you were confused.

This was my first time changing a tire on my own, but I figured, "how hard can it be?" I got out and got the spare tire, the jack, and the lug wrench. All set, or so I thought. Unfortunately, my car was a VW, which means that the lug nuts are not the same ones you would find on domestic cars. They are a different shape, and so they require a special lug wrench, of course. Was I in possession of such a valuable tool? No, I was not. The joys of buying a used car. As a result, I found myself trudging down the side of the highway back to town. It took an hour. The first gas station I found did not have this rare item either. Back to the road. Luckily, the next place I came to had what I needed. Another hour's walk back, and I was all set.

Of course, I didn't make it for the second day either. I was already making a great impression. I was also very hot and sweaty.

The day after that, we began our clinical. For this, we had to travel to another nearby city. Most of us lived elsewhere, so we had to commute. My drive was just over an hour each way. Since most of us did not live nearby, this meant that we were in a totally new environment as well. I had never even been to this hospital before. We spent the first few days just getting ourselves oriented.

The ER where we were doing our training was quite small and rundown. It was only slightly larger than the ER where I worked, but it saw about four times as many patients. There were six of us taking the course, plus our instructor. On each shift, there were also about nine other nurses. It was a bit of a tight squeeze.

What can I say about our instructor? Some people hold vast amounts of knowledge, others are great teachers. Rarely, you find an individual who is both, as he was. He was patient with our limitations, he advocated strongly for us so that we were included in important learning opportunities, and he was honest with us about our mistakes. In the ER, there are many people who are very smart. Many tend to hold that knowledge close to the vest and seem somewhat reluctant to share it. Others wave their intelligence around like a stick. Our instructor willingly shared with us what he knew, and he did it in ways that made it more understandable for us. I cannot recall ever seeing a question that stumped him. I swear that he must have known almost everything there was to know about ER nursing. I worked with him for many years after that, and I don't think a shift ever went by where I did not learn something from him.

During our clinical, something must have clicked inside of me. Up until this point, I had always felt rather daft and more than a bit klutzy. When I started the course, I seemed to find the beginnings of a rhythm for the first time. I still, of course, felt like a novice. However, I began to find a sense of confidence within myself that had been very much lacking up until that point.

The staff, for the most part, were great. It was still a very stressful environment, of course, but the staff seemed happier and more relaxed than the staff at my previous hospital. I was a little bit in awe during those first days. There was so much to take in, but they all helped to make it easier. That's not to imply that it was all great. There are certain nurses who should never be allowed around students, and we had to work with them as well. We got shared around a lot, and we had to go where the action was. As a student, I learned very quickly who was good to work around and who wasn't.

At this point, I should probably clarify something. When I say that certain nurses should not be around students, it's not to say that they were not good nurses. The ER is a very stressful environment, and we all cope in different ways. Some have a need to exert control over the environment, and they hold on to that control very tightly. Others tend to look at students as an inconvenience because we don't know a whole lot and can sometimes get in the way. That attitude can make it very hard to connect with those nurses, and there were some rather uncomfortable shifts as a result.

I was always very relaxed when I was working. Some nurses can just accept the chaos and still function. That is not to imply that I do not have any quirks of my own. For starters, I cope with a dark and wildly inappropriate sense of humor. I also have this weird hang-up about my desk always being tidy. There is never any clutter around my station, and I compulsively tidy everywhere as I go. I love working with students, but woe to the student that makes a mess of my space. The irony is that my house is not tidy at all.

At the end of each week (at least, I think it was the end of the week), we had a classroom day. We also had several assignments that we needed to complete throughout the course. Thankfully, none of these involved losing marks for our APA style or I would have flunked out right away. Most of the assignments were case studies. We would pick a particularly interesting case and present it to the class. We would also have to do further research on the topic, so that we could include all the relevant information in our presentation. I did one on diabetes, with the most complex diagram ever produced. There were arrows and lines going all over the place. I think I probably confused more people than I informed. Despite this, I received high marks for my assignments throughout the course. Afterwards, the woman who had taught us during the classroom sessions told me that she had seriously doubted I would make it at the beginning of the course. After I had missed the first two sessions, she had formed a rather poor opinion of me. By the end, however, she had been quite impressed with my work.

I was about two-thirds of the way into the course when everything went to hell. Now remember, even though I was taking the course, I was still employed by the other hospital. For some reason, my manager decided she was going to pull me out of the course and put me into a new position. I get where she was coming from. There was no way I was going to get a job in the ER afterwards, because they still wanted me to have a few years of floor experience. I really did understand that part. Just let me finish the damn course! I knew that if I left, I would never get back in. I would never have been able to fulfill my dream.

This was all presented to me around lunchtime, and I was expected to show up for work the very next day, ready and willing. I was in total panic mode at this point. Not only had they screwed my career plans entirely, but they had done it in such a way that I had no alternative but to comply. Now you know why I hated that place so much.

When I arrived home that evening, I got a phone call from the manager of the other ER where I was doing the training. Apparently, my instructor had explained my situation to her. She had an open position that she was willing to hire me for, right there and then. Of course, I took it. I then had to go to my old job and tell them that I would not be in the next day for my shift. I was very fond of the nurse who was in charge that night, so I really didn't like putting her in that position. Still, leaving them in the lurch like that was just a little bit satisfying, I must admit.

The next day, I was back in clinical. I finished the course and graduated with honors. Hah!

The year after, there was another newly graduated nurse who was in the same situation I had been in. I guess my leaving had made an impact of some sort. They were reluctant to repeat the same mistake, or to lose another nurse, so she was allowed to go straight from school into the ER course.

WHAT IS THAT SMELL?

Immediately after finishing the course, I started in my new position. In fact, I think I literally only had the weekend off. That was also the weekend that I got married, so everything seemed to be happening a little too fast.

As I stated earlier, there is a big transition from being a student to a nurse. Well, there is an even bigger transition when you start working in the ER. ER nurses have to be just a little bit more knowledgeable than other nurses, so you feel that much dumber by comparison. To be clear, I am not saying that ER nurses are smarter. Nurses in the ER are just very different from other types of nurses. Instead of knowing a lot about one particular subject, we have to know a little about everything because we see every type of problem come through our doors daily.

For my first shift, I had been given the busiest assignment in the department. We had nine monitored spots, split between two nurses. This meant that someone got four patients, and someone got five. Also, the person who had the four beds tended to get more straightforward cardiac patients. The five-bed section was more of a mixed bag of abdominal pains, possible strokes, broken hips, etc. So not only did that assignment have more patients, but there was often more work to do with each patient as well. If I had to say one good thing about that first shift, it is that I didn't have any time to worry about being new. To be frank, I don't think I had time to even breathe.

I remember that one of the beds didn't even have a proper monitor. It had this ancient looking thing, about the size of a small car, that literally looked like one of those computers from the forties. Holding it in place were large metal brackets that were bolted into the wall. The entire setup appeared quite precarious. Not only did the monitor not work very well, but I was certain that one day it was going to fall down and squash one of the patients like a bug. To make matters worse, it was located in the bed that was the farthest from the nursing desk, so it was also the hardest spot to see. It was finally replaced about a year and a half later.

On that note, I suppose I should give you a little verbal tour of the department.

In front we had the monitored spots. These were stretchers with curtains in between. On the side of each stretcher was just enough room for the nurse to stand, if we stood sideways and tried not to breathe. I can recall working a code blue in one of these beds, when I was suddenly bumped from behind. I turned to see a bare bottom coming through a gap in the curtains. It belonged to the patient in the next bed.

There were two nurses working in this area on each shift. Often, we would have contagious patients in this area as well. For instance, we would frequently get patients with pneumonia who would be coughing quite rigorously. No one seemed very concerned that infections might spread, however. Apparently, those curtains were made from some type of super powered cloth that was impervious to germs.

In the back of the department was a long hallway with several rooms. These rooms did not contain monitors, so they were only used for seeing stable patients. By stable, I mean that we were not concerned that their condition would suddenly change. Often, there were at least one or two admitted patients in these rooms as well.

There was also a gynecology room and a lockdown room in this hallway. The gynecology room had a special stretcher with stirrups in place of a regular stretcher. The lockdown room was used for our psychiatric patients. There were two nurses per shift in the back hall. At the beginning of each shift, we would divide up all the patients. Because of our two special rooms, I would often ask my partner if they wanted "coo-coos" or "hoo-hoos".

The most interesting shifts were when we had two male nurses working in the back hall. As a rule, a male physician needed to be accompanied by a female nurse when examining a woman in the gynecology room. This was done to avoid any accusations of sexual misconduct. It also helped to make the patients feel more comfortable. This, of course, presented a problem when there were two guys working back there. If one of the doctors needed to see a patient in the gynecology room, we would be left scrambling for an available female nurse. Being such a busy department, that often involved a bit of a wait until someone was free.

In between the monitored beds and the back hall was a large U-shaped counter. This was utilized as a nurses' station. It wrapped around a central area where we kept things like our photocopier and other such items. The unit clerk had a desk here as well. On the back-hall side of the desk was our medication room and a tiny little kitchen. We spent many a night shift all crammed into that kitchen while we hungrily munched on whatever snacks were available.

Facing toward the front, there was a big entryway on the right-hand side. This was where the ambulance crews would enter. On the far side of the entrance was where our triage desk was located, with a small waiting room on the other side of that. Behind the triage desk, there were two more curtained areas for stretchers.

Across the entrance way and toward the back was the door to our acute room. This was really just a big room that we had designated for traumas. It contained four beds, but one of these beds was reserved for any critical cases that came in. In theory, our code bed was always supposed to be vacant. Reality often interfered with our plans, though. If the department was busy, this bed would often be filled as well. We had to constantly be aware of who could be pulled out, in case we needed an empty spot in a hurry.

Having four stretchers in this room could be problematic at times. I can remember often working on traumas in that room while three other patients were in there as well. We kept the curtains closed, of course, but they could certainly hear everything. This setup also required us to keep an eye on the other three patients, even as we were working to save a life. It was definitely not ideal.

When nurses first started working in the ER, we were restricted to working in the monitored spots or the back hall. As we gained experience, we would then be trained to work in the other areas.

At the back of the big entrance way was a long hallway that led into the hospital proper. About halfway down was a little cupboard that served as our treatment room. Here we saw the walking wounded: people who needed casts or stitches. Simple things. Next to that was another little cupboard that served as our staff room.

Everything in the department looked very old and worn out. The veneer was peeling away from all the wood surfaces. There were cracks in everything. There was almost no light from outside. Oh, and it *always* smelled really bad, as if the normal hospital smell (which is bad enough) had been left to rot somewhere for an extended length of time. Here, we would toil away the hours, trying to keep the people of the city alive for one more day.

...

Our city is kind of a perfect storm when it comes to keeping the ER busy. We have a huge elderly population, a widespread addictions problem (both alcohol and drugs), and a lack of family doctors. In other words, we have a great deal of people with very complex medical needs and nowhere else for them to go. There was rarely a day that we weren't busy.

What made all this tolerable was the staff. In the emergency department we worked as a team, and I'm sure the same is true of all ERs. When you are all crammed into such a small space and it is that busy, you have to work together or else nothing gets accomplished. On most nursing wards, the doctors come in, write a few orders, and leave. The nurses are usually a team, but there's never really much closeness with the physicians. Surgical floors are a little better, but there is still a very clear divide. In the ER and in the ICU, we work with the same doctors, day in and day out. We become a very tight-knit group.

Not to say that we didn't have our moments. Working under pressure all the time takes its toll. Occasionally, staff members would have epic blow-outs. For the most part, however, there was a real team spirit that permeated through everything that we did.

I imagine that this is at least part of the reason they were willing to hire me in the first place, when I was still so fresh out of nursing school. There was always a lot of support there for me, so I was never really alone. To be fair, this level of support would not have been possible at my first hospital. The staffing levels would simply not have allowed for it. This is the main reason why they had been so reluctant to take on new grads in the ER. The dynamic in this hospital allowed for such an arrangement.

I was one of the first nurses in this area to make that transition right out of school. There were two nurses the year before me, and I was the only one from my year. Now, it has become quite a common occurrence, especially in our department.

There have been some studies done on this, and they have found that there are actual benefits to doing it this way. Previously, the thought was that new nurses had to gain floor experience before moving into specialties. They needed to learn what sick looks like. However, the studies showed that there were just as many benefits to taking new grads. The reason is that nurses who have worked on the floors for a few years often develop habits that can be difficult to break. New nurses, in contrast, are easier to mold and have no habits to unlearn. This is because, in the ER, nurses have to be somewhat autonomous. In addition, ER nurses need to have finely honed assessment skills, which means that we are trained to look at specific systems, rather than the patient as a whole. We also have to be fairly comfortable with chaos (in nursing school, we called this the "capacity for ambiguity"). I am not suggesting that floor nurses don't possess these skills or that they can't learn them. It's just that floor nurses get used to a routine, or at least as much of a routine as you get anywhere in nursing. In fact, when I did my course, the nurse who had the greatest difficulty adjusting had fifteen years' experience on the wards. In the ER, there is simply no routine, ever.

I used to joke that there are three types of nurses in the world. New nurses, old nurses, and emergency nurses. New nurses call up the doctor and say, "This is what is wrong with the patient. What would you like me to do?" Old nurses call up the doctor and say, "This is what is wrong with the patient. This is what I want to do about it." Emergency nurses call up the doctor and say, "This is what is wrong with the patient. This is what I have already done to fix the patient. Now I need you to sign off on these orders, ok?"

It's not quite true, but you get the gist of it. Even many of the ICU nurses have trouble making the transition to the ER because of the chaotic atmosphere. Of course, the same is true the other way. I could never work in an ICU because I would never be able to focus on one patient for that long.

If you still can't see the difference, think of it this way. The floors are like a nice family restaurant. A good pace, but there's decent service, and everyone is kept reasonably happy. The ICU is like fine dining. There is lots of individual attention given, and every item on the menu has been perfected. The ER is the McDonald's of health care. We serve it up fast and then we are on to the next. Now imagine what would happen if you took a world class chef and forced them to flip burgers. Not only would the chef be very unhappy with the arrangement, they would, most likely, make a complete cock-up of it as well.

. . .

One thing that I will never forget from my first year of work was the commute. I had gotten married one day before I started the new job, and we still lived in the town where I had gone to college. The drive was about an hour each way. Don't forget that we also worked twelve-hour shifts. That makes for a very long day.

Now, this wasn't all bad. On day shifts, the drive often gave me a chance to mentally prepare for work. I also got a chance to decompress a little on the way back, so that I wasn't carrying my work home with me. It was tiring, to be sure, and it did make the days that much longer. Still, I have always found a certain peace when driving. It's almost meditative for me.

On the other hand, driving home after a night shift was always rough. Being up all night does terrible things to a person's body. It completely messes with the circadian rhythm. Most mornings, I would feel like hell. It's like a hangover, only without the fun night before. It also shaves years off our life expectancies, apparently. I will admit that, more than a few times, I would arrive home in the morning and realize that I didn't remember the drive at all. That's how exhausted I was. I am amazed that I didn't pass out and swerve right into a ditch somewhere.

I was also having some trouble with my car at that point. Yes, the same car that had blown both tires on the first day of the course. Now, the head gasket had cracked, so I was leaking oil everywhere. In order to replace it, the entire motor needs to be removed and then disassembled. At the time, I simply couldn't afford that. Besides, it would have cost more than the car itself was worth. Instead, I would just carry several bottles of oil with me every day. About halfway to work I would have to stop and refill. I would do the same on the way home.

Luckily, we don't get a lot of snow here. I remember one day when it did snow. It didn't look too bad at first, so I set off down the highway as usual. Well, when I was about a quarter of the way to work, it turned into a full-on blizzard. I could barely see anything, and I was travelling along the main highway at 25 kph. About two-thirds of the way there, the highway goes down a fairly steep hill. I had started down, but I was beginning to slide quite a bit, so I applied the brakes. By this point, though, the car had decided that it was just going to keep going. Luckily, I was not travelling very fast as I slid into the roadside barrier. The entire event reminded me of bumper cars. There was a sort of "boink" noise, and the car just kind of bounced right off. Thank God for fiberglass fenders. The snow was deep at this point, so I wasn't going anywhere. Attempts to back up onto the highway proved futile. I was also pretty shaken up by the whole event. That was my first real accident. I called in sick to work, and I resolved to go home once the snowplows had managed to clear the roads, which was about two hours later. The next day, I was informed that snow is not a reason to call in sick. Given how rattled I was, I still think that it was legit.

. . .

The one event that all new ER nurses remember most is their first code blue. I am certainly no exception. I think that I was working in the back hall that day. Suddenly, someone burst into the triage area yelling for help. Apparently, this person had brought a friend down in their van, and the friend was now unconscious. One of the other nurses and I went out to see what was happening. One look told us all that we needed to know. The friend was very near dead, slumped over in the front seat. I remember thinking that he was the same color as Barney the Dinosaur. We managed to get him onto a stretcher and into the acute room. Once there, I started doing CPR while someone else got him all hooked up to the machines. The doctor came in with a resident in tow. Now, as I said, it was obvious that he was too far gone. The resident, however, wanted to save him. As a result, we were forced to continue for quite some time. Eventually, one of the nurses asked if we were going to stop, but the resident still wasn't ready to give up. This seemed a pretty gross violation of the patient's dignity. Don't get me wrong. If there's a chance to save someone, I will bust a gut to do everything possible, and I will not give up. When you are dead, though, you're dead. Anything beyond that is just ego on our part, as far as I am concerned. I took my hands of the chest, exclaimed loudly, "I'm out," and walked away.

Now, I always warn patients to take an ambulance in such circumstances. Here's the thing. Most of those paramedics get paid by the trip. They are just sitting around waiting for your call. That doesn't mean that you should call them for just anything, but some conditions are definitely worth it. They also have a whole bunch of stuff in the back of the ambulance, stuff that can be of some use if your friend happens to pass out on the way. Just saying.

. . .

It was during my first year that I made a very bad decision. At the time, it seemed as though it was a good idea. Now, looking back, I have a "what were you thinking?" moment. The department was short-staffed, so I agreed to come in for a couple of overtime shifts. Well damn, didn't my next paycheck look good. From that point on, I was an addict. I would come in for overtime shifts three or four times every two weeks. I did so much overtime during those first couple of years that I was consistently one of the top five earners for our area. That is a pretty remarkable achievement when you consider that I was at the bottom of the pay scale. At the time, it didn't really feel like a big deal. I had the energy, and the pay was certainly a very nice bonus. At this point in my life, however, I can't help but wonder if that played a role in my current mental state. Maybe I burned myself out. Perhaps if I had not spent so much time there in the beginning, I might still be there today.

. . .

A year after I had started working there, I took a trauma course for nurses. After finishing, I was able to start working in the acute room, which seemed like a pretty big step up at the time. I don't know why, but it made me feel very nervous, like I was going to make a mistake and kill someone. I think that is a common fear for new nurses, and not an unreasonable one, especially in critical care areas where a mistake can have devastating consequences. The irony is that you are more likely to make a mistake when you are nervous, because you start to rush and don't think things through properly. Steps get missed, or nurses don't take the time to really focus on the task at hand. My advice to all the new nurses out there (and the old ones who don't work codes very often) is this: slow down. I know that sounds counterintuitive, but it works.

See, over the years I have come upon a little-known secret. If I have a critically ill patient, and they need something right this very second, it's already too late. They're done. Anything I do at that point is not going to make one tiny bit of difference. Now, this doesn't mean that we should all take our time. There are still tasks that must be done sooner rather than later, so don't get overly relaxed. It is ok, however, to take those extra few seconds. Make sure that you are doing your task correctly. If you have ever watched a video of any special forces units in action, take a moment to really study their movements. They never burst in, guns blazing. They pick a target and fire, pick another target and fire. They all have a saying: "Slow is smooth, and smooth is fast." That means slow down and think, because mistakes cost more time than care does. Say that to yourself during your next code and you will be fine.

I remember once, someone telling me that ER nurses are good in a crisis. I replied that we're not. No one is good *in* a crisis. ER nurses learn to think *around* the crisis instead, if that makes any sense.

Besides, I discovered that the acute room wasn't all that different from any other area of the department. Most of the time, there were just regular patients in there. Over time, I even came to enjoy traumas (well, perhaps "enjoy" isn't the appropriate word there). The truth is traumas are often simpler than other cases. Take a patient with abdominal pain. When I first see the patient, I have no idea what could be causing their discomfort. All ER nurses have little rolodexes in our heads, and we rapidly flip through them for all the possible causes of abdominal pain. Once we come to a likely suspect, we try to order the appropriate tests. Hopefully, we are right. In a trauma, there's no guesswork. They are almost simplistic: everything is done in order, and that order never varies. A trauma takes away the need to figure out what *might* be wrong with the patient.

I believe I mentioned the two-year rule earlier on, and at this point I was still only one year in. I was still pretty shaky. However, I did feel a little better about my nursing, and I had started to gain some real confidence. I did discover that I have a talent for starting IVs. I'm totally bragging here, but I can start an IV on pretty much anyone. I am the guy they call when no one else can get one started. That made me feel pretty good, and it's those little things that really boost new nurses up. I can even remember the first time I got one on a difficult patient. This person had no veins whatsoever, and one of the doctors was about to start a central line. I managed to find one good vein in the patient's thigh and popped the IV right in there. The doctor was not very happy. He had really been looking forward to starting the central line, as he lives for stuff like that. He looked like I had just taken his favorite toy away.

There were even a few patients that would allow only me to start their IVs. In fact, one of them helped me a great deal when I was writing this book.

There were other events that also served to boost my self-esteem. In my life, whenever I have moved to a new area, I never really feel that it is home at first. I feel like an outsider. Then, someone will stop and ask me for directions, and I will know where to direct them. It's that "I've really arrived" moment. This is very true for nurses as well. My moment came when I had an obese patient with a catheter. His belly was constantly drooping down and blocking off the catheter. As a result, he couldn't pee. Well, I grabbed one of our pliable splints (called SAM splints) and set to bending it into shape. I fashioned a little bridge out of it and slipped it over his legs and under his belly. It lifted everything just enough to take the weight off the catheter, and he had no more problems. I figured that if I could come up with a solution like that on the fly, I was ready for anything.

...

After about a year, the new ER nurses must undergo a rite of passage that will test them beyond all reasonable limits. It is now sink or swim time. Only after they have survived this brutal baptism of fire do they truly become part of the fold. We call this experience "triage."

The triage nurse is the person who sits at the front desk and welcomes all who enter. They are the first people you see when you come in, the gatekeepers. They collect all your information and send you on to the appropriate area as quick as can be.

Their job sounds almost easy when expressed in those terms. The reality, of course, is a little different. First off, there are people everywhere, and every single one of them needs to tell you something *right now*! In our department, the triage nurses (there were usually two during the day) were responsible for not only triaging new patients, but also for a host of other things. Behind our desk, there were usually two patients in stretchers. On busy days, there were also a few more patients on stretchers scattered around the entrance area. These were usually patients who needed to lie down but weren't that serious. Broken bones, that sort of thing. They were also the responsibility of the triage nurses. I will tell you, there is nothing that fills me with more joy than knowing that all the patients in my care are receiving such undivided attention. Yeah, that never really happened. With a steady stream of patients coming in the front door, we rarely had time to look at the patients behind us. Often, doctors' orders for things like pain medication could sit for quite a while, until one of us had an opportunity to get to them. To complicate matters further, these patients were people, with people-like needs. I used to get a very special feeling in my gut whenever I was busy triaging someone, while the patient directly behind me used the commode. The sound effects alone really added something special to the experience.

That is not even the end of it. Oh no. We were also responsible for all the patients in the waiting room. These are the people who have been triaged but haven't gotten a spot inside yet. It was expected that we would go out and check on them and do vitals, on a regular basis. That didn't happen very often, either.

Then there's the actual triaging. We had two lines of patients to deal with, those walking in and those coming in by ambulance. We would listen to their stories and then assign them triage levels based on how acute they were. That triage level would determine where they went within the department and how quickly they would be sent there. Level one means that this person needs attention right now. Level five means that the patient probably needs a band-aid and a tetanus shot.

Now, I realize that a lot of the people reading this are probably "in the biz." For those of you that aren't, let me clear up some things for you. Triage is not like the deli or the bank. There is no number system. It is not first come, first served. The sickest people go to the front of the line. That's just the way it's done. This is why we have a big red sign over the front door that says "Emergency."

On one particular occasion, I had just finished triaging a patient, so I took a second to scan the waiting room. There was a guy who was coming in through the front door and he looked absolutely awful, all pale and pasty. He was looking at the lineup in front of him with some dismay, obviously concerned about the wait. I pointed directly at him. "You, you're next," I said. You should have heard the rumblings from the other people waiting. It turned out that the patient was bleeding internally, so I had made the right call.

The reality is that I am quite good at my job. I can spot sick very well. In fact, I am so good at spotting sick people that I easily manage to avoid them on my days off. That way, I don't end up having to perform CPR in the grocery store. For this reason, trying to make it sound like you are sicker than you actually are will not get you seen faster. I know you're feeling miserable, but I can pretty much guarantee that you are going to survive. I will often tell patients that waiting is a good thing because it means that we are not that worried about you. It's the people who don't have to wait at all that need to be concerned. The one thing you never want is for the ER staff to get excited by your arrival. That never leads to good things. That does not mean that we don't make mistakes, so if anything changes you should come up and tell us immediately. Otherwise, please, just wait your turn.

Also, coming by ambulance will not get you seen faster. Not only that, if you take an ambulance off the street when someone else might really need one, you will not incur my goodwill. This was one of my greatest pet peeves when I worked there.

Last, please give people some privacy. I cannot even tell you how many times I have had patients telling me the most intimate details of their lives, while some stranger insists on standing two feet behind them. People stand further back than that at Tim Hortons, for God's sake. Just give people the same amount of space that you would want them to give you, once it is your turn.

There, that's my rant. I can hear triage nurses everywhere yelling out their thanks. You're welcome.

By far the best aspect of working triage (warning, sarcasm ahead) is that we become the face of the department. In fact, we must be personally responsible for the failures of the whole damn system. I cannot count the number of times that I have been yelled at, called names, threatened, and even assaulted. I am not a small guy, but I have had people literally come at me over the triage desk. I can't even imagine what some of the female nurses must go through.

There was an incident where one of our triage nurses actually got punched in the face, just because a new arrival felt that he was not being dealt with fast enough. The worst part is that the nurse was told, by management, that it was really all his fault. He must have done something to aggravate the person who assaulted him.

Yes, triage can be a very exciting place to work.

Of course, just when it seems that you have a handle on triage, they throw yet another curveball at you. This one is called "charge." I was about two years in the first time I was put in charge of the department. Let me tell you, it was a real eye-opener. When we work as regular nurses, we are only responsible for our little piece of the puzzle. I think that we all develop a bit of tunnel vision, myself included. Whatever my problem is at that moment, it is the most important problem of all. Everyone else's problems will just have to wait. Once we are put in charge, suddenly we are responsible for the whole department. Everyone's problems suddenly become my problems, and every single nurse will insist that their problems are the priority.

I should mention that there were a few full-time charge nurses, but they were only present for the day shifts. At night, or when there was no regular charge nurse scheduled, they would pick one of the senior staff instead. At some later date, the full-time charge nurses were put on a rotation that included night shifts. After that, we would only have to be in charge occasionally, such as when we covered vacation or sick days. I did charge a great deal.

Most of what the charge nurse does is flow. As I mentioned earlier, the ER is like the McDonald's of health care. We rely on getting people in and seen quickly, and that means getting them out just as fast. Every bed occupied by a patient is a bed we can't use for a new patient. The person in charge has to try and facilitate that movement. We need the patients to go elsewhere—either home or to a room within the hospital, if they are admitted. It sounds a great deal easier than it is. Usually, once they are admitted, there is nowhere else for them to go. Our hospital often runs at over 100 percent capacity. Most of my day as charge was spent having people tell me why they *couldn't* help me, or what they *couldn't* do for me.

Often, even the people being sent home can present a challenge. Sometimes the patients are elderly, and we have to ensure that they are getting home safely. This can entail keeping them in a bed until we are able to arrange suitable transportation. We also had a policy that we would never send elderly patients home at night if they lived alone. Other times, we have patients who are not elderly but still have no way of getting home. You would be amazed at just how many adults arrive at the hospital with no plans for leaving once they are seen and discharged.

Me: Do you have family?

Patient: No.

Me: Do you have friends?

Patient: No.

Me: How were you planning on getting home?

Patient: I assumed that the hospital would be taking care of that.

To be clear. Our job is to get you to the hospital (by ambulance) and then to fix you. After that, you are basically on your own. Figure it out.

The worst feeling in the world is being in charge and having a department full of inpatients. There is a deep sense of dread that settles in the gut because there is simply no place to go. When that happens, it means that people coming in have to wait, which basically entails sacrificing the safety of unstable new patients in favor of stable admitted patients. Somehow this scenario makes sense to the powers that be. Often, people can spend a few days in the ER waiting for a bed on the wards, especially if they need a bed in a specialty area, like telemetry. There were days when I was positive we would end up running a code blue on the park bench out front, simply because there was no room inside.

I will say this for the ER: we suck at inpatient care. It's not because we are bad nurses. It's simply that inpatients are never our priority. Often, they will get their medications as scheduled. After that, we will pop in on them every few hours just to make sure they don't need anything. Otherwise, we generally ignore them. We simply do not have the time to provide them with any extras, which they do receive on the floors. Simple things, like a warm washcloth in the morning, become luxuries that we simply don't have time for.

There is one thing that we can always count on with inpatients. For some unknown reason, every single one of them will have to pee at the same time.

Usually at the worst possible moment. A new patient will come in having a heart attack, and every single call bell in the place will suddenly light up. It's like they all wait specifically for the most inconvenient time. I have also found that elderly people, especially women, all appear to have bladders the size of walnuts. Thus, they will routinely have to sit on the commode once every ten minutes, like clockwork. Then, there is the 4 a.m. rule. All elderly patients will wake up and have to pee at 4 a.m., without fail. This used to drive me crazy. Now, as I get older, I find myself in the same boat.

I also find it funny that, despite the hospital always being full, the admitting clerks are still required to ask patients if they would like to pay extra for a private room. Like we have any of those available, ever. When we do, they almost always have to be earmarked for patients who may be contagious. Some days, we are so overcrowded that patients are lucky they still have a private bed. We may just end up making everyone spoon one day in the near future.

One of the reasons that we are so full all the time is the fact that we still operate like a small-town hospital, even as our city expands. This means that most of our specialists go home at night. Essentially, much of the hospital only functions nine-to-five. The specialists are still on call, and they do get paid to be on call. Woe to anyone who actually does call them, however. To be fair, only a few of them are really like that. Sometimes we can't get patients sent upstairs at night, even if there are beds, simply because the specialists are not there to write admission orders.

I recall one patient who had yanked out his catheter at home. He was bleeding quite profusely and our efforts to stop it were not successful. The urologist at the time refused to come in, stating that, "There's no such thing as a urology emergency." In the end, the patient continued to bleed and ended up in the ICU. Seemed like a urology emergency to me.

It's not only the physicians, either. I like to joke that we must be the only hospital in the world where the coffee shop has better hours than the pharmacy. It sounds funny, but it's not.

Another charge nurse job involves looking after all the other nurses and their needs. Some days, unfortunately, it can be a little like running a daycare. I say this with all the love in the world, but sometimes my fellow nurses can be just a little needy. When I first started working in the ER, I can remember looking at the other nurses as almost godlike. That impression faded quickly once I had done a few charge shifts. People would be coming to me with problems that they could easily have fixed themselves. Often, I would end up playing referee if there was a personality conflict. I had people tell me that they had not been able to take their breaks, ten hours into a shift (when it is too late to do anything). By far, my favorite was when we were short-staffed, and nurses would demand that I send help to their area. Contrary to what they might have thought, I did not have an extra staff member hidden up my butt.

I can remember one time when the department was absolutely packed to the rafters, leaving us without a single monitored spot. I came up with a pretty radical solution to fix the situation, and one of the nurses didn't like it at all. She just kept yelling at me, "You can't do that. You can't do that." Finally, I turned around and asked what her solution would be. She just stared at me blankly. We did it my way, and it got us through the night.

To do all these different jobs, the charge nurse needs to carry around a phone at all times. This phone is specifically designed to ring once every five minutes, throughout the entire shift. Some days, it is almost impossible to do anything other than answer the damn phone. To this day, I still have indentations on my ear from the speaker. I did get very skilled at holding it between my ear and my shoulder, however. So much so that my neck will no longer bend all the way to the right. Now there's a talent I can put on my resume.

Still, being in charge could be very rewarding at times. One day, I received a phone call from the paramedics. They informed me that they were coming to us with an infant in cardiac arrest. In ten minutes, I had everyone ready to go. I called pediatrics and had them send a nurse down. I also had a psychiatric nurse standing by to counsel the family if they needed it. Unfortunately, once the baby arrived, we very quickly realized that there was nothing we could do. I think we only worked at it for about ten minutes or so before we stopped.

Afterwards, I gathered everyone together just to check in. I made sure that everyone was ok. The primary nurse was a brand-new father, so I insisted that he go home for a while to see his own child. Then, I spent some time with the family, consoling them. I always feel very proud about how I handled that case.

...

At this point, we averaged 130 patients per day. That is a lot of patients to see when we only had twenty-three stretchers in the department. The rest of the patients would have to take a seat in the waiting room, sometimes for hours on end. As I stated earlier, there was often no time to check up on them as they waited.

Because of these factors, our department was forced to find innovative solutions. We instituted several firsts in our department, simply because we had to. There was just no other way to deal with that kind of volume.

We implemented something called streaming. This became imperative after we had a patient die in our waiting room, simply because no one had checked on him in hours. It was decided that patients would be far better off getting into the department right away, where the nurses could keep an eye on them at least. They would still be waiting, but it was now supervised waiting.

In order to facilitate this, we removed most of the beds in the back hall. The only ones that remained were in the gynecology and psych rooms because we still needed those. Our largest room was converted into a waiting area, and all the others were to be used as exam rooms. Instead of having people lie down in beds, we had patients sit in chairs until they could be seen. They would then be taken to one of the exam rooms, seen by a doctor, and taken right back to the waiting room.

We also developed several protocols, which allowed the nurses to order tests on the patients as soon as they arrived. Tests no longer had to wait until after patients were seen by a doctor. This way, the results were available as soon as the doctor was ready. Patients could then be sent home or admitted immediately after the doctor had examined them.

We also developed a pain protocol, so we could start providing medication to the patients right away. When the doctors did see them, many patients were already pain free. This also allowed them to be sent home quickly.

Of course, this meant that only patients who were able to sit could go there. It certainly did create a great deal more room for patients. We could now have thirty patients in the back hall, instead of eight. No more patients waiting out in front of the triage desk where no one would be able to look at them.

The monitored beds remained as they were.

All in all, this idea worked really well. Many of the nurses were not very happy about streaming at first. The triage nurse no longer had to look after all those patients, but the back-hall nurses now did. It meant that we could have up to fifteen patients per nurse back there, which is way too many for one nurse to look after effectively. What made it better was that each patient had been looked over by someone, and they were always visible now. It was safer than it had been. I always looked at it as a bad solution for an even worse problem.

Not that this did not create new problems. There was one patient who got very sick after a few visits. When I looked at my charting from one of his visits, there was only an initial assessment done. The rest of the chart was totally blank. What saved my ass was that I could prove just how busy I had been that day. I can usually keep track of up to twelve patients. After twelve, I have to write the diagnosis down or I will forget. There, in one corner of the chart, was such a notation.

Another case involved a young man who had come in with what had seemed to be a minor complaint. He was sent to the back hall and put into one of the exam rooms. I can't remember who it was that went to check on him later, but he was out cold, face down on the counter. We quickly rushed him out to one of the monitored spots, and one of the doctors came to intubate him. Well, things quickly went from bad to worse. He ended up in ICU, where he passed away later in the day. We all felt bad about this case. I seriously doubt that the outcome would have changed had he gone straight to a monitored bed, but I don't know that for certain.

The biggest problem with streaming was that we became quite good at it. Sometimes, I really think that we are our own worst enemies. We went from having long wait times to having some of the shortest wait times in the country. In fact, our wait times were so low that people started coming in droves. We quickly became the best show in town. As a result, our numbers climbed sharply, and we became just as crowded as we had been before streaming.

...

While all of this was happening, another event of great significance occurred. I took on my first student nurse. She was in her fourth year and was studying at the local university. In the ER, we will only take fourth year students because only they will have enough knowledge to make the experience worthwhile. In such a complex environment, third year students would be very limited in what they could do because they would lack the necessary understanding.

Because I absolutely love teaching, I was very excited to have a student. Unfortunately, it did not go at all as I had envisioned. The truth is, I think she was very intimidated by the staff and the ER in general. From the very beginning, she kept talking about how dumb she felt. I tried my best to reassure her. In the end, she spent all her time looking after the admitted patients instead. She even had one of the medical nurses take over as her preceptor. I really regret the fact that I didn't prepare her better, as I thought that she was a very good nurse. I hope at some point she managed to explore the ER further, wherever she ended up working.

As a result of that experience, I now tell every student I work with the same thing. No one expects them to be ER nurses at this point. Instead, I expect them to perform like reasonably competent fourth year students. That is my only expectation.

. . .

It was also around this time that my marriage fell apart. Now, I certainly don't think that this was all my fault. However, I contributed to it. I am what I like to call an introverted extrovert. That means that I can act like I am extroverted at work, but it is not my natural demeanor. As a result, I would basically come home and just clam up. I needed time to recharge, and to do that I needed quiet. There's no way a marriage can survive that. I have since learned that this is a common occupational hazard. To all the poor souls reading this, if you are married to a nurse, you have my undying sympathy.

. . .

There was something else that happened during this period. I began to notice that whenever I was in charge, I would often end up having to phone the police because one of our psych patients had escaped. This kept happening because the nurses felt it was cruel to leave the patients locked up all the time. Now, I don't disagree. It is cruel. It is also much safer. Often, we would leave the door open if the patient was well behaved. What I would often tell the nurses is that, in psychiatric patients, previous behavior can never be used to predict future behavior. That is the very essence of psychiatric illnesses. Because of this, I became very active in educating the staff about psychiatric patients and their conditions. I would also do workshops with the new nurses. I did a great deal of research on the subject, so I really knew my stuff. I would take every opportunity I could to pass that knowledge along. We still had some escapes after that, but not as many.

· · ·

Perhaps one of my favorite jobs of all was going on transfers. This is when we have to take a patient to another hospital, usually because they need a service that we don't offer at our facility. We are a mid-level hospital. This means that we act as a hub of sorts. Smaller local hospitals send more complicated patients to us. We, in turn, have to send critical patients to the larger centers. We stabilize as best we can, and then send the patients on.

Sometimes the patients can go with just the paramedics. However, if they are unstable, they need to be accompanied by someone more qualified. We sometimes have the option to fly them out by helicopter, if they are really ill. The choppers are staffed by paramedics with advanced training. There is also a critical care ambulance that is available for transfers, but only during the day. Often, if neither of these options are available, a nurse must go. Hopefully, that nurse would be me.

There were other times when the patient was stable but needed some sort of medication that the regular paramedics couldn't give. For instance, I had to transfer a psych patient once. He was a big guy, so the paramedics were concerned about safety. The paramedics wanted to keep him sedated the whole way, so I went along to administer the sedation.

I will say that we are highly trained for this, so that we know exactly what to do in case the patient goes downhill. I have been very lucky in this regard. I have done a lot of transfers, and only once have I even had cause for alarm. Even in that case, nothing actually happened. I did make the ambulance speed up and turn on the siren, though. The truth is, if it ever came right down to it, I am never going to try and run a code blue in the back of an ambulance. I am not even certain that the defibrillator would work properly, given all the motion. They often cannot tell the difference between a bump on the road and an arrhythmia. While on transfers, we are never more than fifteen minutes from some sort of medical facility anyway. In such a circumstance, I would perform CPR and tell the crew to head for one of those facilities, fast. Realistically, that would give the patient a much better chance anyway.

Most of the time, transfers are very routine; I basically sit there and do nothing for the entire trip. Every so often, I have to write down vitals or give an injection, but that's about it. On the way back, it's even better. You can grab a pretty decent snooze because you're all alone in the back. There's even a stretcher to lie down on.

I also love talking to the paramedics during transfers. They might not have the same training that we do, but they are consummate professionals nonetheless. Truth be told, I could never do their job. Just trying to give IV meds as we are bouncing down the highway can be challenging enough. I have great respect and admiration for everything the paramedics do. For starters, they see the patients in way worse shape than we ever do. It's their job to scrape the patients off the highway and bring them to us. Sometimes, in order to get a patient, they have to enter homes that are just packed with refuse. Paramedics deserve a hell of a lot more respect than they are given, especially by our current health care system.

Sometimes, there can be a lot of screwups along the way. Ambulance dispatch is in charge of telling the ambulance crews where to go. I often get the distinct impression that they have no idea what is going on out there in the real world. Once, I was transporting a very sick patient. He had several IV pumps going, and I had to take the portable defibrillator with us as well. Dispatch actually sent me an ambulance that was broken. There was no electricity available at all. I had all these machines that needed to be plugged in and no power. To make things worse, we didn't have time to wait around for another ambulance, so I had to make do. The portable defibrillators have enough juice on their own for one, possibly two shocks. Any more than that and an outside power supply is needed, much like what we would have access to, had we been able to plug the damn thing in!

Then, there was another thing that really made me angry. Often, the dispatch people would send us ambulances from some of the smaller communities. This was done in order to save money. The arrangement worked out great on the way down. However, this often meant that they could only come back as far as their home station. They would then have to kick us out, and we would be forced to make our own way back to the hospital.

I got into a heated argument with one of the dispatchers over this. As far as I can see, we are doing them a favor. The ambulance service is mandated to transport patients, not us. We go along because, in order to keep costs down, they are not provided with the resources they need to fulfill that mandate. Kicking us out on the side of the highway is a pretty shoddy way of thanking us for helping them. It also leaves the ER short-staffed for a longer period of time. Not to mention the cab fare costs. I have frequently taken cab rides costing $150 or more.

On one transfer, dispatch ordered the paramedics to kick me out because the crew had to do another transfer. It turned out that the other transfer ended up going to my hospital anyway. They arrived back before I did.

Another time, there was an admitted patient who needed to go to a nearby hospital for a procedure. He had a few medications running, so they needed a critical care nurse to go with him. The patient and I were all ready to go, when the crew began loading a second patient into the ambulance. He was going to the same place, so dispatch had figured, "why not take him as well?" I will tell you why not. If I am going with a patient, there is a reason for that. I am there in case things go wrong. Should things go wrong, I would need space to work. Besides, how would it look to the other patient if the guy I was taking suddenly crashed right next to him? No one wants to see me working a code blue on someone less than a foot away. Hell, I would probably have a heart attack right there if I was that person. Also, who wants my butt in their face as I'm doing CPR? The entire situation was completely absurd, and I flat out refused to allow it.

...

After I had been working for about two years, we hired a new department manager. She was great in many ways, but a little odd in her management style. She definitely played favorites. If she liked you, you were in. She would go out of her way to be there for you. If she didn't like you, nothing you could do was ever going to be right. I was lucky. I was in the first group.

I had a good friend of mine who was most definitely *not* in the first group. She was a new grad, and she looked after our overnight patients. As someone who was in charge a lot, I really enjoyed working with her because she always went above and beyond. I could call her to take a patient and she was one of the few who would never argue about it. If we were busy, she would even come and grab the patient herself. She never complained about how hard the work was, she just got it done.

For some reason, the manager absolutely hated her. This nurse had to go in for knee surgery, and the manager decided that she was faking the whole thing. I knew she wasn't because I had taken her in on the day of her surgery. My friend was so intimidated and afraid of losing her job that she returned to work far too early. She could still barely move her leg. This backfired as the manager now decided that she was just lazy. The manager essentially hounded her until she quit. Then, once my friend had left her position, the manager also went after her nursing license. It was the most vindictive and petty thing I have ever seen a manager do. Not liking someone in no way justifies ruining their life like that.

I am a very smart person. I know it. When I say that, though, I don't mean to brag. It's more of an awareness. The reality is, I don't see it as an accomplishment. I didn't earn it in any way. It's not like God saw fit to reward me for some great deed I had performed. It was an accident, a fluke of genetics. It's like being attractive. No one has any say in it.

There are some people, however, who forget just how smart they are. These people start setting really high standards for others, and then look down on those people when they can't live up to those expectations. It's intellectual snobbery. This manager was like that.

She was an enormous influence for change in our department. She had a real vision for how we could improve our delivery of care. Many of these changes were completely radical and new. It helped that the Chief of Emergency Medicine at the time possessed an almost identical temperament. Streaming had been one of their innovations, for example.

The problem was, neither of them possessed the patience to deal with the naysayers. There are always going to be those who have difficulty adjusting to change, and those people need to be supported and coaxed along. Instead, the manager and chief would ram the changes through, and then browbeat the naysayers until they complied. It gets the job done, but it certainly doesn't endear a manager to those who work for them.

Several years later, they both played a part in the biggest debacle we ever had in the hospital, but I'll get to that later. This is where such a personality type can become a real drawback. When you assume that you are so much smarter than others, it becomes almost impossible to accept and acknowledge your own mistakes. Objectivity is lost, and people can get steamrolled in the process.

. . .

There is one last thing that I should probably tell you about myself, before I finish out this chapter. I absolutely hate being the center of attention. There is something called imposter syndrome. It is the feeling of being an outsider, or that one is not deserving of success. Some people, like me, have it worse than others. Now, this doesn't mean that I lack confidence. It is more the belief that I am somehow different, that I don't really belong. Perhaps it is an expectation that *others* will not recognize my competence. Consistently, I feel as if someone is going to come up to me at any moment, tap me on the shoulder, and say, "We know about you! You're not supposed to be here." I am fine when people criticize me. In fact, I welcome it. I believe that criticism gives me a chance to grow and learn. However, when someone pays me a compliment, I don't know how to take it. Praise makes me feel very uncomfortable. I will usually try to make my escape as quickly as possible. This is the reason why, in all my years as an ER nurse, not one person has ever learned when my birthday is (and I'm certainly not about to tell you either). Just the thought of having people sing "Happy Birthday" to me gives me shivers. It is a real shame, because I absolutely love eating cake.

SHITS AND GIGGLES

Ok, I wasn't going to do this. I told you how much I despise war stories. There are some stories, however, that just have to be told. See, the crew that I work with are the most hard-working and dedicated people I have ever met. Of course, this doesn't mean that we don't have our moments. We make mistakes just like everyone else. Some of these stories are funny, and some are quite tragic. They have all affected us in some way. These are the stories that we end up carrying around with us for the rest of our careers.

Just think of this chapter as our blooper reel.

One of my favorite stories occurred about a year after I started working there. I was in the back hall, and I was working with one of my favorite nurses. Now, I have mentioned that I'm not a small guy. The woman I was working with was probably even tougher than me. I can't recall exactly how, but our psych patient managed to get himself out of the lockdown room. My partner and I immediately tackled him to the ground, and it took both of us to hold him there. As I mentioned, neither of us is little, so you can just imagine how hard this guy was struggling. He was positively superhuman. To make matters worse, he had gotten hold of a syringe as we were taking him down and was then trying very hard to stab us with it.

Into the fray stepped another nurse who had come to our aid. Now, this other nurse has been working in the ER for a very long time. She is a wonderful person and one of the smartest people I know. She is also as by-the-book as they come. So, there we all are. The two of us are struggling with all our might to keep this guy pinned down. Meanwhile, the other nurse has brought us a shot of medication to sedate him. I watched as she carefully took the back of his jeans down. Then, she opened up her alcohol swab and began wiping his buttocks with very precise circles. It was all so delicate. At that point, of course, my partner and I are screaming, "Just stick it in! Just stick it in!" Eventually she gave him the shot, but she made damn sure it was all done properly. Had it been me, that needle would have been jabbed right through his clothing.

...

Most of the time, we will work very hard to save a life. Sometimes, however, we have to know when to stop, when a situation has become hopeless. I will give you a good example. I once had a patient who had come in because he had been ill for several weeks. His family had come in with him, and they had essentially forced him to come to the hospital (yes, he was one of THOSE guys). All in all, he seemed in good spirits, but the family was obviously nervous as they stood at his bedside. I was certain that the family was right to be concerned. Given his symptoms, I knew that the diagnosis was not going to be a good one. The patient didn't seem to get this, but the family certainly had their suspicions. Still, he didn't appear to be in any imminent danger, so I tried to engage with the family in order to reassure them. I told them that I thought this might be serious, but that I had no immediate concerns about his safety. My talk worked, as the family appeared calmer.

After a while, the doctor came in and ordered a CT scan. Obviously, we needed to get a clearer picture of what was going on inside the patient and what had caused him to become so ill. I was about to wheel him over to medical imaging, so the family decided that this would be a good time to go for lunch. Based on what I had told them, they were no longer concerned about leaving him for a short period of time. Since the CT scan would take a while anyway, this would be a perfect time for them to eat. We went for the scan, and they went down to the cafeteria.

When we returned from medical imaging, the patient was sitting up in bed and chatting away. Suddenly, he coughed, and everything went straight to hell. This is not an exaggeration. I had to roll him up onto his side immediately in order to keep his airway open. Unfortunately, in this position, I could not reach the code blue button to call for help. The gods must have been looking down on me because another nurse picked that precise moment to enter the room. I had her push the button and help quickly arrived.

We worked on that guy for a solid hour, I think. Half of the staff was in the room, and we were all doing everything we could. It was pure chaos, and the entire room looked as if a giant bomb had exploded. However, in the end, nothing we did was working. He was slipping away too fast for us to keep up. As I said, we will fight to the bitter end when it's appropriate. In this case, it was now obvious that the time had come to give up, which is what we did.

The worst part was that I had sent the family off. I had assured them that nothing was going to happen right away. Of course, they had returned from lunch in the middle of all this. They walked in on what can only be described as an utter disaster. I felt really guilty about that, which is why I have included the story here. They had left feeling reassured and had returned to a scene that resembled a horror film. There was a look of complete shock on their faces.

I also felt bad for the other patients in the room. Remember, our acute room did not have anything that even resembled privacy. As soon as help arrived, my first words were, "Get all of these people out of here, now!" The charge nurse grabbed each of them in turn and wheeled them away. I have no idea where she actually put them, as we were completely full that day. Even though we had managed to get them out quickly, what they did manage to see must have been quite traumatizing for them.

...

At one time, we had a doctor working in our department who is pretty much a legend within the ER community. He has worked everywhere and has probably forgotten more than many of us will ever learn in our lifetimes. The crazy thing is, he was also the epitome of the absent-minded professor. He would often be seen roaming the department, muttering under his breath as he searched for some item that he had just misplaced. Whenever he would write orders on a chart, he would often just hand the chart to whoever was standing closest to him at the time. Sometimes, that happened to be a nurse, but other times it could just as easily have been one of the housekeepers. I am not meaning this to be an insult, by the way. All his quirks were actually sort of charming.

On this particular occasion, I had gone on break and another nurse was watching my section. When I returned, I could see that this doctor was standing beside one of my patients. One of the nurses was standing on the other side of the bed watching the monitor, which displayed the patient's heart rhythm. On the monitor, everything looked good. The problem was, neither of them appeared to have looked at the actual patient. From across the room, I could tell that things were very wrong. The patient had lost any semblance of color and didn't appear to be breathing. I sprinted across the room and grabbed for his neck, trying to find a pulse. Of course, it wasn't there. Some cardiac arrests are what we call PEA arrests, which stands for pulseless electrical activity. The heart is still getting signals to beat but isn't actually doing anything. Sometimes the heart is not contracting properly, and sometimes it is, but there is simply no blood to pump around. On the heart monitor, of course, everything looked fine. I started CPR immediately, but it was unsuccessful. The patient ended up passing away a few minutes later.

I always use this story with students, because it illustrates a very important point. "Treat the patient, not the machine." The monitor is only a tool. Those numbers mean absolutely nothing unless we know how to interpret them in the context of what is actually happening for the patient.

I just remember how the doctor and nurse looked when I had come back. They both were standing there like they didn't have a care in the world.

...

One quality that I really admire about our team is just how dedicated they all are. It was Christmas day, and the ER was very busy. Suddenly, this guy came running in carrying his little terrier who had apparently just choked on a chicken ball. I have no idea why he was feeding his dog chicken balls for Christmas dinner. Anyway, damned if one of our doctors didn't grab that dog, place it on top of one of the tables, and go to work. One of our advanced care paramedics jumped in, and they valiantly attempted to intubate the poor pooch. Unfortunately, that chicken ball was solidly wedged in there, so they were unsuccessful. Still, it was a pretty heroic effort on their part, and all because they didn't want this poor guy to lose his dog at Christmas time.

...

There is one nurse who has been with the department for a long time. Almost as long as I have. He is an amazing nurse, but I swear that he can fall asleep anywhere. We were on a night shift and he had just returned from break. As soon as he came back, he vanished. No one could figure out where he had gone, and we ended up searching the department for him. In the end, we found him asleep on one of the stretchers in the monitored area. He had crawled in there and closed the curtains, so everyone had just assumed that there was a patient in there.

Another time, I found him asleep again. He was actually lying across the desk in the acute room.

. . .

Once, I was in charge on a night shift when my computer suddenly crashed. To be an effective charge nurse, we need the computer. Without it, we are totally blind to what is going on in the department, so it's kind of a big deal when it stops working like that. When I attempted to start the computer up again, I got a message on the screen that said that such-and-such error had occurred. It advised that I should go to this certain website for more information. Now, just think about that for a second. "I would love to visit your website so that I can fix my computer. Unfortunately, I really need my computer to visit your web site." It was kind of a catch-22 situation, if you ask me.

. . .

After my first experience with a nursing student, I really wanted to try again, since things had gone so badly. This time, I went out of my way to pick a student that I knew would be good. I really wanted someone who would be easy to teach, so I approached one of our student nurses and offered to be her preceptor. I had picked well, and she grew into a very talented nurse. There was one event, however, that still makes me laugh. We had a patient who was quite intoxicated. He was also agitated and violent, so we were trying very hard to restrain him. While we were holding him as still as possible, my student attempted to start an IV. I was holding his arm up above his head. I guess that this position threw her orientation off, because she was trying very hard to start an IV in the wrong direction (IVs always point towards the heart). She will probably punch me for including that story.

...

One of the things that is unique to working in the ER is what we call our "frequent fliers." These are the people who come in day after day, for whatever reason. Now, you will often hear us grumble when they come in, simply because we see them so often. This can get on our nerves, since we are so busy already. However, when you work in the ER, a strange thing happens. They can start to become like family. Now, when I say family, I am probably talking about the crazy uncle that no one likes to talk about. Still, family nonetheless.

There was one of these patients who would be brought in every single day. She was a hard-core alcoholic and was also homeless. Often, she would pass out on the grass, and some well-meaning passerby would phone the ambulance for her. The ironic thing is that she didn't want to come to the hospital. She was quite happy sleeping on the grass, right where she was.

After seeing her every shift for almost two years, she suddenly passed away. This was the first time that I had experienced the loss of one of our frequent fliers. I was surprised to find that I really felt the loss. I think we all did. From that day on, I have refused to treat our frequent fliers with any less dignity than our other patients. They deserve our respect as well.

Another one of our frequent fliers was a guy who had a lot of psychiatric issues. He would always cause quite a ruckus when he came in, but he was quite harmless. Well, one day he came in screaming his head off about something. This was, of course, done in the middle of a very crowded waiting room, so all the other people were quite horrified. I am sure that they thought he was dying. It took a great deal of time to get him calmed down so that we could find out what had happened. It turned out that he had stepped on his pet at home and was worried that he had injured it. What had appeared to be a life-and-death emergency at first turned out to be something very minor.

...

I am sure that there are a lot of people who still think nurses don't do very much. They assume that we are only there to follow the doctors around, doing whatever they say. What everyone needs to realize is just how smart the nurses actually are, and just how often we save the patients from mistakes the doctors have made. I can't tell you how many times that has happened to me. Now, this is not to say that we have a bunch of bad doctors. It's just that they are human, like the rest of us. When you are seeing thirty to forty patients in a shift, errors are bound to creep in. Once, a doctor wanted me to give a medication, but called out the oral dose instead of the IV dose, which was much smaller than the oral dose. One of our new people had started drawing it up, not realizing the error. Thankfully, I managed to intercept the new nurse and correct the dose before we killed the patient.

Often, we will get orders for antibiotics that the patient is allergic to. Sometimes, they write the correct order on the wrong chart. On occasion, I have seen them misplace a decimal point. Errors do happen sometimes. Because the nurses know their stuff, we are able to avoid such errors as they occur.

I can remember once getting an order for "nitro patch SL." Now, let me explain. First off, for those of you that are unfamiliar, nitroglycerin is a medication that we often give to cardiac patients to relieve chest pain. SL means sub-lingual, or under the tongue. This is what we do with nitro pills or spray. I am sure you can appreciate that a nitro *patch* (that goes on the skin) would probably leave quite a foul taste in your mouth, were I to try and shove it under your tongue.

On another occasion, I had a patient who was having a heart attack. Now, most of the time these patients can benefit from nitroglycerin, but sometimes it can kill them. This happens when a patient's heart is not able to contract with enough strength to maintain blood pressure, because the nitro will lower the BP even further. I have had several patients over the years like this, and many still get orders for nitro spray. The physicians often write the order simply out of habit.

Whenever patients were kept overnight, we had a special room for them to stay in. We also had printed order sets for the most common cases, so that the doctors would not have to write out the orders each time. One such order set was for patients who had overdosed on Tylenol. Now, many of you are probably thinking, "Tylenol?" Well, believe it or not, an overdose of Tylenol can be deadly. It completely pooches (yes, that's the medical term) your liver. To counteract it, we have to give the patient an infusion of a drug called acetylcysteine, which requires several hours to complete. Anyway, back to the point of the story. On the printed orders for a Tylenol overdose it said, "For pain, give Tylenol." It was a standard order on all the order sets, so someone had just copied it without thinking. Perhaps an order for some other type of pain medication would have been more appropriate.

...

There is an ICU doctor in our hospital who is famous for his lengthy orders. He is one of the smartest people that I have ever met, and he can figure out what is wrong with just about anybody. He is our hospital's Dr. House. Unfortunately, this means that he will usually request every test he can think of for his patients. As a result, his orders often resemble *War and Peace*, with a really long introduction and that extra-large type they use for people who can't see very well. There is nothing like the look a new nurse gets on their face the first time they have one of his patients. Their eyes go blank with shock as they peruse the fifty-page order before them. One nurse in our department basically laid it out for him. "If you want it to get done in the ER, it better be on the first page."

It so happens that another one of our ICU doctors is a man of few words. Correction, a man of *very* few words. In twelve years, I think I could count on my fingers the number of times I have heard him speak. I doubt that I have ever heard a complete sentence from him. Every year, he would send us a Christmas card, and all it would say was Merry Christmas and his name. That was it. On one shift, one of the ICU nurses had to call him for an order. After explaining what was going on with the patient, the nurse stopped talking and waited for a reply. There was silence on the other end, and the nurse quipped, "I think that asshole hung up on me." Then came the terse reply: "No, the asshole is thinking."

There was an incident, once, where one of our ER doctors was in the middle of a very long shift. He was talking to a psychiatric patient who was telling the doctor that no one ever listened to him. He looked over and the doctor had actually fallen fast asleep. I know, this sounds made up, but it's true.

...

One thing that doctors will often include in their orders is IV fluid. They include what kind of fluid (we actually have several different kinds, despite what they show on TV), as well as an exact rate to run it at. I am always trying to tell them that we don't really do rates in the ER. There's fast, slow, and somewhere in the middle.

In fact, I describe ER nurses as the masters of "ish." Everything that we do is measured by "ish." Twenty-ish milliliters, one hundred-ish kilograms. You get the idea. We don't do exact in the ER, most of the time. We tend to live in the gray areas.

. . .

I recall one time that I was in charge, and we had a patient locked up in the psych room. He was none too happy about being locked up, of course. In order to exact his revenge on us, he had blocked the door so that no one could get in. We called security, and they spent about ten minutes discussing various plans. None seemed particularly viable. One of the security guys even suggested that he crawl through the ceiling. After ten minutes, I was fed up with this whole scene. I walked up to the door and said, "Look, we are going to get in there. How angry we are when we do get in is entirely dependent on how long it takes us." I must have sounded very serious, because he immediately began to dismantle his makeshift blockade.

. . .

Perhaps the strangest incident that I can remember occurred on one of my night shifts. Our overnight doctor was due to arrive at any moment, and I just knew that it was going to be an interesting night. For some reason, whenever I was on shift with this particular doctor, some bizarre event would befall us. He just had that kind of karma (he still works there too). Anyway, there was an emergency generator test scheduled for that night. The main power was turned off, and the emergency generator came on as expected. However, when they switched back to main power, it came back on everywhere in the hospital but the ER. No one could figure out why, so it took the maintenance guys several hours to restore power to us. As a result, when our night doc arrived, we were all sitting there in absolute darkness. I did mention that there were no windows, right? Luckily, we are a clever bunch, so we managed to make do. We had all the patients on battery operated monitors. We also managed to gather up every flashlight in the building. I can still recall holding the flashlight very steady as one of the lab techs tried to take blood from one of the patients. As luck would have it, we ended up having a very slow shift that night. To this day, I believe that this is because our "emergency" sign was on the same circuit as the rest of the department, so it was also dark. People probably just assumed that we were closed.

...

I am certainly not going to leave myself out of the fun, so here are a couple of my own less than stellar moments. For starters, one day I was working at triage when a patient arrived by ambulance. He had fallen and broken a bone. I was pretty busy, so I didn't really look at the patient. The paramedics didn't tell me anything that would have alarmed me either. Just a story of what had happened. Well, I directed the ambulance to unload the patient onto a stretcher. Just then, I saw one of the doctors sprinting toward the triage desk, as fast as he could run. What I hadn't noticed (and what the paramedics didn't mention) was that the affected limb was pointing in the wrong direction. It was also very blue. If we had left that for too long, he would have lost the limb due to lack of circulation. I always lay eyes on the patient now, no matter what the paramedics tell me.

In the last chapter, I talked about the problem of psychiatric patients escaping. Well, even I made that mistake once or twice. I was trying to be nice to one patient and I had left the door open for her. Of course, as soon as my back was turned, she was off. The funny thing is, she called us about twenty minutes later to apologize for leaving, and also to let us know that she was fine. She was afraid that we would be worried about her. Call display is such a wonderful thing. I did a reverse lookup of the number and was able to provide the police with her exact location. They had her in custody again about fifteen minutes later.

There was a night where I was assisting with a code blue on one of the floors. The patient was in critical condition, so the doctor and I were working very hard. The biggest struggle for me had been to get an IV going. Her veins were so flat that even I was having a great deal of difficulty. After trying multiple times, I finally managed to get one in. About fifteen minutes later, I accidently tripped over the IV tubing and pulled the entire thing out. We were back to square one. I told you that I'm a klutz.

...

You may be wondering why I am telling you all these stories. Partly because I want you to be entertained. Partly to allow you a glimpse into our lives and a chance to read about the experiences that help us to grow as nurses and doctors. I also include them to make a very important point. See, people who work in the medical field tend to have alpha personalities. We are driven and more than a little bossy. Also, we are quite often perfectionists, and we will hold ourselves accountable to a fault. Many times, getting off work, I would run through the events of the day. It was never my successes that I would end up obsessing over. It was always the mistakes. Big or small, they would keep me up at night. I would incessantly pick at them while I stared at the ceiling until 3 a.m. This is the case for most of the nurses and doctors that I know. It is even more true in critical care areas. As a result, it is no surprise that our mental health is at risk sometimes. We carry guilt and shame around with us constantly, and that can have deadly consequences.

During my third year on the job, one of our co-workers committed suicide after making an error. This is very common. In fact, suicide rates among health care professionals are twice as high as they are in the general population. Unfortunately, because of our training, suicide attempts are almost always successful in health care professionals. We know *exactly* what to do.

IT'S ALL FUN AND GAMES UNTIL SOMEONE LOSES THEIR HEALTH CARE

D espite the title, I have deliberately avoided humor in this chapter. Some things just aren't funny.

This chapter is all about what I think is wrong with our health care system. I am including this so that you can better understand my experiences and the circumstances that led up to my current condition. Most of the issues that I talk about contribute significantly to the level of stress experienced by health care workers. As such, they relate directly to our emotional well-being. Keep in mind that what follows is only my opinion. I have only anecdotal evidence to back most of this up, so take everything I say with a grain of salt.

If you happen to reside in a different country, I hope that you will still read this chapter. I am certain that many of these factors are present everywhere, so you may still find it useful and educational.

For starters, let me state right off the bat that I am a firm believer in a publicly funded system. There is no argument that anyone could ever make that would convince me of the need for private medical care. Our system has its problems, and it is very far from perfect, but it is also a far better system than most.

What I do not believe in is a system that is also publicly run. When a system is run by the public (via our politicians), that system ends up setting priorities that are based on public perception rather than on medical needs. Politicians are loath to make unpopular decisions, even when those decisions are based on actual science and research.

I will give you a perfect example of this. We have known for decades that addiction is a mental health issue. Every single addict out there suffers from some form of mental illness, either diagnosed or undiagnosed. They are what we call self-medicators. We also know that giving addicts access to services, such as safe injection sites, needle exchanges, placement in rehabilitation, expanded mental health services, and safe housing, saves us money in the long run. It saves us in policing costs, crime reduction, insurance payouts, and emergency services. Despite all the evidence, people still cling to the belief that addiction is a choice. They think that people just wake up one morning and say, "I want to be a drug addict." People with addiction issues are seen as dirty, or as criminals who deserve whatever fate befalls them. As a result, the public doesn't want to "waste" money on them. One appalling fact is that, in my city, there are presently very few rehab beds available. Patients have to wait weeks to access them. By taking the public's opinion out of the equation, we could actually reduce costs. And this is only the first example.

A second great example is emergency rooms. ER overcrowding is one of those hot-button issues that always gets people fired up. This is because ERs are the public face of health care. They remain the access point for a lot of people. What people see is how overcrowded ERs can become. They have to wait for hours sometimes, and this makes them angry. For this reason, ERs have become the focus of public spending. We end up building new emergency rooms or upgrading old ones. The problem is that ERs are not really the cause of overcrowding. We are the middle ground between the community systems and the hospital systems. Lack of services in either of these areas is what actually produces overcrowding. Unable to see a family doctor, come to the emergency room. Unable to access home care or other community services, again, come to the emergency room. In the hospital, lack of space and resources on the wards mean that patients have to remain in the emergency department for longer periods of time. In other words, emergency departments are overcrowded because of inadequacies in other areas.

When we built the new ER at my hospital, one of the surgeons summed it up perfectly: "It's like putting a bigger funnel on the same size hose."

However, because ER overcrowding is what people see, that's what gets the funding.

This becomes an even bigger problem when you consider that emergency rooms, being an acute care area, are one of the more expensive parts of the health care system. The fact that we have also turned them into one of the most efficient areas (in terms of getting people seen and treated) is just not cost-effective. It means that the price of accessing care costs a great deal more because patients are forced to access costlier areas when cheaper alternatives are not made available to them.

Beside our triage desk is a price list for ER services. This is meant for people who come in from somewhere else, like tourists who do not have coverage. A lot of times, when local people see this list, they will comment on how lucky we are in this country because we don't have to pay. The reality is that we *do* have to pay, just not up front. That is what it costs when anyone comes to us for care. If a patient accesses the ER for something that they could have seen their family doctor for, it actually costs the system approximately ten times the amount of money.

All too often, this is the route that many patients are forced into. With the lack of family doctors, where are they supposed to go for medical care. There is also a lack of walk-in clinics for minor complaints, and where they do exist, the hours often prohibit working people from being able to attend.

I am in no way trying to suggest that people should not come to the ER when they need to. I am simply saying that we need to get away from this idea that shoveling more money at emergency rooms is going to help. It is not a viable or sustainable solution. If people can't access family doctors, fix *that* problem instead.

Yet another example of wasteful spending is how we manage care homes for the elderly. Older people are another group that society has turned its back on, and that is atrocious. Because of our views on the elderly, our government started to privatize their care many years ago. Many care homes are now privately operated. This means that profit margins must be maintained, even at the expense of patient care. The result is that they often understaff these facilities. There can sometimes be one RN who is responsible for the care of every resident, with the bulk of the staff being made up of (cheaper) care aides. This is not to disparage the work of the care aides in any way. They are hard workers and are the unsung heroes of the health care system. They do not, however, possess the training to properly assess and diagnose the residents under their care. As a result, potential problems may get overlooked. Also, when a resident does become ill, these facilities are often unwilling to absorb the cost of providing adequate care. So when a resident gets sick, they are sent to hospital. The public system must then absorb the cost, and this care is far costlier than if we had provided them with the same care in the home.

We will often get inpatients with dementia from the care homes who are quite agitated. Due to poorly trained staff, these patients are a danger to themselves and to others. As a result, they are sent to us. Guess what happens when you take a patient with dementia and place them in an unfamiliar environment, especially when it is very noisy? They become even more agitated because they are frightened. All we can do is load them up with drugs and send them back.

I have even seen patients come in from care homes with blocked catheters. This takes about two minutes to fix, but it is a procedure that must be done by a nurse. If there is no nurse available at the care home, these patients also get sent to the ER. When I worked there, I would sometimes not even triage those patients. I would take them somewhere private, give the catheter a good flush while they were still on the ambulance cot, and then turn them right around.

I have also come to believe that we, as a society, are very reluctant to talk about dying. That is an impression that has stayed with me throughout my career. I am amazed at how many people want us to do absolutely everything to save them, no matter how hopeless it is. It's not that I think we should never try to save the elderly, but I do believe that people (especially the elderly) need to be properly informed when it comes to the subject of resuscitation. It's not like on TV, where the hero pushes on the chest twice and the patient immediately sits up, totally cured, and walks out of the hospital two days later. In real life it is brutal and often long. We break ribs, we stick tubes everywhere, and we zap you with electricity over and over. Often, we can't bring people back no matter what we do. Unlike TV, we often can't even use the defibrillator because it will not work on the patient's particular heart rhythm (anyone flat lining is a perfect example). When we can save someone, it can sometimes be worse than if we had allowed them to pass. Brain damage is common, due to lack of oxygen. Needless to say, the elderly suffer the most and have the least chance of recovery. Please, if you take nothing else away with you after reading this book, talk to your loved ones. Be frank and know the facts. Make sure you know the wishes of your loved ones, and make sure that they know your wishes.

Now, I am in no way suggesting that we should not respect people's wishes. What I am saying is that those wishes need to be based on sound information rather than false hopes. Patients and families need to be properly informed if they are to make realistic decisions. We also need to discuss our wishes with loved ones *before* we get sick, so that decisions are not being made when emotions are running high.

In case you are wondering, I have a do-not-resuscitate order. I am not even that old, but I have seen what it looks like. I never want anyone doing that to me.

...

The current health care system is what my parents would have called penny-wise and pound-foolish. Our efforts to save money cost us far more in the long run. To keep taxpayers happy, budgets are intentionally lowballed based on the best-case scenario. This approach is not realistic because the best-case scenario *never* happens. If people need to access the system, they are going to access the system. If they are sick, they are going to come to the hospital, whether all our beds are full or not. They don't care, and they shouldn't have to.

You might remember way back when I mentioned my job in the restaurant. Just like my old boss, the health care system is obsessed with saving every penny. Sometimes, however, cutting costs can create significant inefficiencies.

Currently, my employer is already millions of dollars over-budget and we are only into August. The bulk of this is because of huge overtime costs as we attempt to cover for higher patient volumes. More patients means we need more nurses. It's simple math. Then there's the need to replace nurses who call in sick because of burnout or stress.

Many nurses simply choose to leave the profession. Others, like me, are forced to leave. Then we not only have to bear the cost of covering their shifts, but there is also the added cost of training replacements. It can cost up to $100,000 to train a new nurse. My story is a perfect example of this. It certainly doesn't have to be.

All these costs add up very quickly. We end up spending way more than we would have if we had just paid for adequate staffing levels to begin with. We need to start budgeting for the worst-case scenario, not the best.

In the emergency department, understaffing can become very problematic. Often, we are only hanging on by a thread to begin with. High patient volumes mean that the staff is spread thin, and this leaves us unable to respond adequately to contingencies. All it takes is a trauma or two to arrive, and everything else comes grinding to a complete halt. The severely injured must always be our highest priority. Inadequate staffing levels decrease our ability to respond appropriately when an actual emergency does come in. It also reduces our ability to provide adequate care to our other patients. Just because someone is currently stable does not mean that they will remain so. The nurses that remain behind in an area while others respond to the trauma may miss signs that a patient is declining because they are now looking after too many people. Emergencies also reduce the number of physicians available to deal with other patients, which results in longer wait times. This increases the risk that these other patients will decline as they wait.

There was a quote that I heard recently: "Inadequate staffing is like drunk driving. Sometimes everyone still gets home ok. However, every single time, lives are put at risk."

I have no first-hand experience, but I am certain that conditions are just as bad on the floors. One thing that the statistics clearly show is that inadequate staffing levels on the wards result in poorer outcomes for patients. Fewer nurses means that patients do not receive the same level of care. If patients are not mobilized often, their recovery takes longer. Not repositioning patients as often results in more bed sores. Infection rates go up. Complications get missed. Every single one of these factors can increase the chance that the patients will have to extend their stay in hospital.

Overcrowding and understaffing also means that patients can sometimes get discharged too soon. When hospitals are over capacity, the pressure falls on staff to discharge as many patients as they can. These patients often decline and end up coming right back again.

This is all just in the hospital. Things are even worse in the community. Increasing funding for home care services is one of the cheapest and most effective ways to fix many of the problems that we face. Again, public perception keeps us from exploring this route to its full potential.

There is still the idea that sick people belong in the hospital. The reality is that the hospital is the last place we should be putting most people, especially the elderly. Why? Because the hospital is where all the sick people are.

Every so often, a patient will get some form of illness while in the hospital. This illness then spreads like a wildfire throughout the entire facility. Patients who are packed in like sardines are more likely to come into direct contact with each other, which makes the spread of infections that much more likely. In a way, hospitals are like perfect little incubators for so many diseases.

C. difficile is a prime example of this. C. diff is what we call an opportunistic infection. It is caused by bacteria that is often already present in the intestines of patients. It is kept in check by the other types of bacteria that also call our intestines home. A good round of antibiotics kills off all the good bacteria, allowing the C. diff to suddenly flourish and spread. It is also highly contagious, and once a case is identified, it has often already spread to others. This happens quite often, especially in the care homes.

Influenza, pneumonia, and other such infections also happen with alarming frequency.

There are other reasons to avoid the hospital as well. Often, I will hear family members talk about how full of life grandpa and grandma are. How they like to hike every day or are active in other ways. At home they were the epitome of healthy living. Here's the thing, though. It doesn't matter how healthy they are. Every eighty-year-old is eighty years old once they get hurt or sick. The minute that they are admitted to hospital, they begin to decline. Lying in a hospital bed swiftly reduces muscle mass, resulting in the loss of mobility. This can happen at the rate of up to 10 percent per day. Their bodies are tired, and they simply lack the metabolic resources to replace what is lost, no matter how healthy they used to be. The end result is that grandma, who used to walk five miles every day, gets discharged from hospital and is suddenly unable to do her own dishes. Guess what happens then? Back to the hospital, where they decline even more. The result is a total and permanent loss of independence.

If you think that I am exaggerating here, consider this. Inpatients over seventy years old who fracture a hip have a one-year mortality rate between 14% and 27.5% (Schnell et al.). For something that is so easily remedied, that number is simply unacceptable and undefendable.

Anyone who has ever been a patient in hospital, or a nurse for that matter, knows just how noisy the environment can be. Lack of sleep also contributes to poorer outcomes, yet patients are constantly woken throughout the night. Sometimes this is because we need to run tests, or perhaps they need medications in the wee hours. Sometimes it's just because their neighbor is having problems sleeping or is doing poorly.

In addition, family can play a very important role in healing. Having loved ones present is of significant benefit to patients, and there are many studies to back this up. In hospitals, the family can only be present at certain times. There may also be limits on how many family members can visit at one time. At home, none of these restrictions are present.

For all patients, but particularly for the elderly, hospitals are the last place to stay if they are to heal. This means that home care needs to be expanded. I would go so far as to say that for every nurse in the hospital, there should be a nurse in home care. Patients cared for at home are less likely to develop debilitating infections. They are more likely to mobilize frequently. They get more rest. Just being in a familiar environment reduces stress and increases the rate of healing. The quicker patients are sent home, the better. But to do this, there must be adequate care in place at home, and that care needs to be consistent.

Nowhere do I see the tragedy of this more often than in palliative care. I am heartbroken by how often I see patients who want to die at home being brought in to the hospital because the family is simply overwhelmed. At other times, they may be lacking in such basics as adequate pain control. As a result, instead of passing in their own bed, they get to die in a hallway somewhere. I have even had patients pass away in the elevators. This could be avoided if they had proper access to resources at home.

Imagine a world where this was a possibility. We could sharply reduce the cost of building and maintaining hospitals. Yes, they would still need to exist. Being at home is simply not a possibility for some. Others may need aids to their recovery, such as equipment or diagnostics, that would simply not be available at home. However, even if we managed to get only some of the patients home in a timelier fashion, the savings would still be enormous.

The most important cost saving measure we could ever implement is public education. In our society, we are brought up with completely unrealistic expectations when it comes to our health.

The internet has vastly increased our access to information, yet so much of it is unreliable at best and totally inaccurate at worst. We need to provide people with the tools that they need to discern the difference between information that is accurate and information that is pure hogwash. I cannot tell you how often I have had people come up to me at triage and say things like, "The internet says that I'm having a stroke." No, you're not. In the hospital, we call this Doctor Google.

The public needs to realize the simple truth that sometimes we get sick. Commercials for cough syrups, cold remedies, this pill, that pill have left society with the belief that there is an instant cure for everything. All a person needs is the magic pill and they will be instantly healed. Sometimes, however, the best cure really is to just stay in bed for a few days. You will feel like crap. That is normal. With a few notable exceptions, most people do not require an emergency room visit for the flu.

Another common misconception people get from TV is that medicine is like some form of magic. On medical shows, the physician will look at a single X-ray and immediately diagnose some rare disease. Then the patient is miraculously cured the next day. That is not how it works in real life. The unpleasant truth is that diagnosing is really just a guess. That's right, a guess. To be totally accurate, it is an educated guess based on scientifically proved methods, but it is a guess nonetheless. That may be unsettling to hear, but there you have it. If it makes you feel any better, most doctors are pretty clever and will usually guess right.

That being said, sometimes a guess is all we have. Sometimes we simply don't have the information available to provide more. Abdominal pain is one thing that can be troublesome to diagnose, particularly when it is chronic. Some conditions are very easy to diagnose, such as gallstones or an inflamed appendix. Other conditions that result in diffuse abdominal pain can be very hard to diagnose. The nerves within the abdominal cavity function rather poorly, so there is often no correlation between where the pain is felt and where it might actually be coming from.

Crohn's disease is a good example of this. Often, patients can become increasingly frustrated as they wait for their doctors to figure out what is causing their pain. Then, people will come in to the emergency room seeking a second opinion. Unfortunately, we often don't know either, and all we can do is make you feel a little better. This is also likely to be counterproductive. Believe it or not, your family doctor is really the best person to see for these conditions. That's because family doctors act like a hub. Information from many different sources, such as diagnostic tests and specialist consults, all flow into one location. This makes diagnosing your condition much easier because all the information is stored in one place. It also increases continuity of care, as your family doctor knows you far better than we ever will in the ER. For all these reasons, they are able to coordinate treatment in a way that will benefit you the most. If you present to the emergency room, we have to start right back at the beginning.

One other thing we can do to reduce costs is to reduce the liability of information centers for the public. In my area, we have a phone number that people can call to get pertinent health information. Numerous studies have found that these helplines do absolutely nothing to reduce costs. People will often call having already decided that they are going to the hospital and are only looking for validation. The people who work in these call centers are so afraid of litigation that they have rigid rules preventing them from advising these patients not to go to the hospital, even when common sense says that it isn't necessary.

Shortness of breath is one of the symptoms that raises red flags for helplines. Yet, our definition of shortness of breath and the patient's definition can be vastly different sometimes. So many times, I will hear patients describe themselves as short of breath. "No, you are congested." Not being able to breath is a very different sensation from feeling stuffy. Just ask any patient with Chronic Obstructive Pulmonary Disease. They will tell you. Yet, if a patient states they are short of breath, the only advice that the helpline can give is to go to the hospital.

Last, but certainly not least, management needs to start listening to the people who work for them. The doctors, the nurses, the care aides, etc. These are the people who are in the trenches every single day. They are your front line. They can tell you what works and what doesn't work, sometimes with annoying clarity. Ignore them at your peril.

I fully realize that all bureaucracies are inefficient by nature, but there are still so many things that we can improve upon. These improvements would not only cut costs, but they would also provide for better patient outcomes and greater patient satisfaction. All it would really take is the political will to do so.

Now back to our regularly scheduled programming.

IT'S SO SHINY

After I had been at my job for three years, we moved ourselves into a new department. It had become increasingly obvious that we had outgrown our little ER, so they had built us a brand spankin' new one. It was state of the art. Instead of being divided by curtains, each stretcher was in a separate room with closing doors. Finally, we were able to isolate people who came in with infectious diseases, such as pneumonia. Patients had privacy as well. We could now talk to our patients without their neighbors overhearing every word.

Also, someone had the foresight to get new monitors. In the old department, our monitors were different from the ones in telemetry and ICU. As a result, every time we moved a patient to one of the other units, all that data was lost. Now, they were compatible with the other monitors in the hospital. The doctors and nurses could now follow all the patient's vital signs and heart rhythms, from the moment they arrived until they were discharged home.

For those with more serious infections, we also had two rooms specifically designed for infection control. These are called negative pressure rooms. When the door is opened to the outside, air is sucked into the room, causing the air pressure within the room to be kept just below the air pressure outside it. As a result, air already inside the room cannot escape. Any viruses or bacteria are therefore trapped. These rooms also have an independent ventilation system, which contains diseases that are able to survive in the air for short periods of time, such as tuberculosis (most diseases, such as the flu, require a surface, such as skin, to survive).

The new trauma bay was impressive as well. There were two pods, which meant that we could handle more than one trauma at a time. In theory, each pod could manage up to four patients. Realistically, we only had room for one patient at each pod. Two, if we really pushed it. It was also a dedicated trauma room, so no more having other patients in there as well (at least, that was the plan).

There was also a large area for streaming, with a huge waiting room and several exam rooms. We now referred to this as the ambulatory area. There was an exam table in each room, much like you would see at a doctor's office. This helped to dissuade patients from getting too comfortable, so that it would be easier to move them back to the waiting room after they had been seen. The first rule of streaming is to never let the patient lie down because you will never get them up again.

There was an enclosed area right next to the nurses' desk that contained four recliners. Here, patients who would be staying for longer could at least get comfortable and put their feet up. This included patients that were waiting for test results or getting IV medications. One of our nurses worked in streaming all the time, so this area was named after her when she retired.

Next to the streaming area, we had a treatment area for minor injuries. This was for patients that had presented needing stitches or with a broken bone that would need casting. One big complaint we had in the old department was that some of these patients required sedation. This was common with dislocations or when a limb required traction before casting. Whenever this situation occurred, the patient would have to be moved to a monitored bed because patients who are sedated tend to hold their breath occasionally. In the new department, the treatment area had three exam rooms, and each room had its own monitor. Patients would no longer be required to move before being sedated. This wasn't always easy, however. Because this area was specifically for minor wounds, patients tended to be seen and discharged quickly. A sedation could tie up the nurse for half an hour, which was hard to deal with in such a fast-paced environment.

We also had our own X-ray room in the department, with a dedicated X-ray technician. Right beside it was a room for doing ECGs. No more having to send people elsewhere to get diagnostics done. The lab also had its own area, and requisitions for blood work would print up there. This helped to streamline the entire process, making everything much faster.

Perhaps the best thing of all, though, was that we now had a psychiatric ER called a PES unit. This was a completely separate area located just down the hall from the main ER, and it was staffed with proper psychiatric nurses. Now, patients with psychiatric complaints could be sent down the hall to this new area, where they would be under the care of nurses with the appropriate training. There was also a lock on the entrance, so patients were allowed to wander free within the confines of the PES. No more being locked in a tiny cell all day, for most of the patients. There were two locked rooms down there for those that posed too great a risk to wander free. The unit even had a small courtyard with a waterfall.

There was quite a lot of discussion during the planning stages for this new area. The psychiatrists wanted to have total control over the unit, which caused quite a few misunderstandings in the beginning. The conversation went something like this.

Psychiatrists: "Well, how many patients will we be taking?"

ER: "I don't understand."

Psychiatrists: "What is the maximum number of patients you will be sending to us?"

ER: "No, you don't understand. This is an emergency room, so there is no maximum."

Psychiatrists: "We are thinking six patients."

ER: "Six patients?"

Psychiatrists: "Yes, six at a time."

ER: "No, again, there is no maximum. You have to take whoever comes in."

I have found that this concept can be very hard to understand for nurses that have never worked in an emergency room. We do not *ever* get to say no in the ER. There is no maximum for us, and we don't turn people away (well, hardly ever). The patients come in and we see them, every last one.

In the end, it was decided that the psychiatric nurses would staff the new unit, but that the ER doctors would initially assess the patients. Anyone that required more attention would then be passed on to the psychiatrists the next day. Also, any patient with medical needs, such as suspected overdoses or patients needing IV medications, would still be held in the main department until medically cleared. After the patient was cleared to go to the PES, we would call down a report. Their first question was always, "Is the patient walkie-talkie (walking and talking)?" This led me to coin the term "stumbly-mumbly," which seemed more appropriate sometimes.

All children would be seen in the main department, unless the PES unit agreed to take them beforehand. Usually, they would not agree if they had any adult patients at the time. This was done to protect the children from being exposed to possible dangers.

The last exception was elderly patients with dementia. They would also have to remain with us. For this purpose, we still had one room with a lock on the door. Occasionally, if our locked room already contained a patient, and we asked really nicely, the PES would agree to take a patient with dementia from us.

There were two rooms used only for sitting down. These rooms were designed for visitors who had a family member in the trauma room. The visitors could sit in there and have the door closed, so that they did not have to listen to all the commotion. We had also found them quite handy for other uses. We would often put our pediatric psych patients into one of these rooms so that they would have a quiet environment to wait in. Then, they would not get over-stimulated or agitated. They were also great for when staff members come in as patients. That way, we don't have to be sitting in the waiting room with all the other people. Membership does have its privileges. This has been especially useful to me over the last couple of years, for reasons I will soon explain.

The last improvement was a dedicated shower room with its own door to the outside. Because of this, patients who were contaminated with chemicals no longer had to travel through the department. They could go right into this room and be rinsed off. This was a vast improvement, as we often got patients who had been pepper-sprayed. When they would arrive in the old department, everyone's eyes would sting for hours.

All in all, the new department was a godsend. Everything had been designed for efficiency. The staff had been given an opportunity to provide feedback before the plans had been finalized, and everything had a natural flow to it. Each room had supplies that were tucked into drawers located right next to the stretchers. There was equipment for starting IVs, gowns for patients, towels, oxygen masks, etc. When we needed these supplies, they were close at hand. For those items that were not in the drawers, we also had a new person whose sole job it was to get us what we needed.

Of course, there were a few problems as well. For instance, in order to save money, the floors had not been properly sealed along the seams. Within a month, they had started to bubble and to peel up at the edges.

There was also a problem with the ventilation system. During construction, the design team had decided to go with thermal heating. This consisted of using a series of tunnels in the basement, designed to draw up the earth's natural heat. As a result, this system requires no power. It was *supposed* to keep us warm in the winter and cool in the summer. In reality, it mostly did the opposite.

I thought that the funniest mistakes were in the new PES area. The nurses' station was supposed to be totally secure so that they could retreat inside if a patient ever became violent. Unfortunately, someone had placed one of the locks on the *outside* of the glass barrier, so any patient would be able to open it easily and gain access. Also, the outside wall with the waterfall had been built too low. Patients were able to climb up on the wall and escape when we first opened.

The ambulance entrance was located directly behind the triage desk. Beside that, there was a large sliding door leading into the trauma room. This was a great addition because it allowed the ambulance crews to take critical patients right inside. Unfortunately, it also afforded every person in the lobby with a great view of whatever might be happening in there.

Also located behind the triage desk was a sink with an eye wash station. Someone had accidentally hooked it directly into the hot water instead of the cold. Anyone using it at that point would have had their eyeballs melted.

To add to the flaws, someone had designed the ER so that it could not sustain any additional weight. Nothing could be built on top of it. There are plans now to build a new ICU, and placing it on top of the ER would have worked very well. No chance of that now. I believe the plan is to build it in the parking lot behind the new ER instead, so it will still be close.

Perhaps the biggest complaint I have heard from staff members was that we might have made the new department too large. In the old department, we had all worked in very close quarters. Now, each area was self-contained, which left the staff feeling somewhat isolated. In the area with the monitored beds, there was a large barrier right in the middle. This only served to increase the feeling of separation because it effectively divided up the entire section. We couldn't see our co-workers on the other side.

Of course, the one drawback of moving into a new department is the move itself. I was off that night, which I am eternally thankful for. In the wee hours of the morning, all the patients had to be packed up and moved over. In addition, all the equipment had to be moved as well. It was a pretty hectic morning, I am certain.

I was on the next night, but by then things had more or less settled down. We still had no idea where anything was, but we did manage to muddle through.

...

For some reason, management had decided that immediately after we moved, we would be switching over to a brand-new computer system. Never throw two new things at your staff at the same time. It's just asking for trouble. Realizing what a disaster it was going to be, I had cleverly arranged my vacation to coincide with this little event. After my two night-shifts, I was off for almost a month.

Predictably, the department was transformed into an absolute madhouse. Our wait times apparently doubled during that first month. As I had hoped, most of the kinks had been worked out by the time I returned.

There is also that old saying, "build it and they will come." When a new ER gets built, people will come in just to see it, rather than going to their doctors' offices. It's like a field trip. Our numbers instantly climbed, and we were full up again within days. I remember running into the Chief of Emergency Medicine in the changeroom after work. At this point, we had only been in the new department for a few months. I asked him, "Now that we have outgrown this department, when will we be building the new department?" He just looked at me with resignation, said "shut up" in a very sulky voice, and walked out.

All in all, it probably took us about six months to really settle in. During this time, we went through one of our big turnovers. These are periods where several senior staff members leave. They never seem to leave one at a time. Some didn't like all the changes. Some were just done and decided that this was a good time to go elsewhere or to retire. Still others moved on to other jobs. For whatever reason, it did create a gap in the expertise level of the staff. I remember looking around one day and realizing that I was no longer the newbie. I was senior staff now. That was a little disconcerting for me.

After the first few months, our numbers began to decline. The novelty of the new department had worn off for the public. This made settling in a great deal easier. Also, the staff were becoming more familiar with the new computer system. As a result, our wait times improved significantly. We were back on top.

...

Shortly after the move into the new department, my ex finally finished nursing school. She began working in the psychiatry department in the same hospital (not the PES, but where the admitted patients are). We started hanging out again during our breaks. I should mention that we had remained in touch throughout her schooling. Since I had already been through the course, I would often be up at her place to help her with assignments and such. Lucky me. It was like going through nursing school twice. I had also continued to support her financially during this time.

On one such occasion, I had gone to her house to help with a big project. She was having a great deal of difficulty with the assignment and was getting increasingly frustrated. At one point, she went on a twenty-minute rant about how much she hated the project, as well as the nursing school in general. I just watched in silence. Once she had calmed down, I pointed out that it didn't matter how much she hated it. The assignment still needed to get done. We got back to work. To all the nursing students out there, remember this little bit of advice. The only way to get through nursing school is to get it done. Jump through whatever hoops you have to jump through. It will seem horrible at the time, but the end is so worth it.

Anyway, I digress. After spending some time together at work, we decided that it would be worth it to try and live together again. In the end, I think we did this for entirely the wrong reasons. I believe that neither of us wanted to be alone anymore. That's never a good reason to be married. We ended up getting a small house together outside of town. I was back to commuting.

She soon found herself unable to work as a nurse any longer. I ended up supporting her for the next three years.

...

One of our regular charge nurses (and one of my greatest mentors) had a daughter who was just entering her fourth year of nursing school. The daughter came to me one day and asked if I was interested in being her preceptor. Apparently, her mother had recommended me. I was a little skeptical at first. I knew that she was very smart, but I wasn't sure exactly how our personality differences would play out. I believe that students learn better when they are placed with preceptors who are not only smart, but also have similar temperaments. I am a bit old and cynical. She was young and bursting with positive energy. It was grumpy bear meets the energizer bunny. Still, once she started her practicum, we worked very well together.

She was indeed very smart. She also seemed to have an instinctive grasp of what it meant to work in the ER. There was still much to learn, but I never felt the need to instruct her on *how* to do the work. I just filled in some of the details.

I remember the first time she had a dying patient. She was visibly upset and had started to cry. I took her aside and told her that tears were for later. Right now, the patient had to come first. She cleaned herself up and went back into the room. For the rest of that experience she behaved like a pro. This isn't to say that nurses shouldn't be able to express our own emotions. Quite the contrary. We should be showing them way more than we actually do. However, when dealing with patients, we have to put those emotions aside. Our patients come first, and the family needs to see us as solid so that they can have a chance to grieve. We can cry, but we have to do it on our own time and out of sight.

Toward the end of her practicum, we experienced one of the worst days I have ever had in the department. A co-worker came in as a patient, and he was very ill. Unfortunately, it was very hard to figure out what was wrong with him. To make matters worse, once he was admitted none of the specialists would take him as a patient. Each of them insisted that it would be more appropriate for someone else to look after him. This is common sometimes in smaller hospitals. It happens when patients are too sick for one service, but *not sick enough* for another service. The end result was that we could not get anyone to write orders for us, even for pain medication. I doubt that I have ever been that frustrated before. My student and I spent over two hours on the phone, haranguing anyone we could think of. Eventually, we got one of the specialists to write up some orders. I think he only did so in the hopes that we would stop calling him.

My student and I became great friends afterwards, despite the differences in our personalities. I even attended her graduation from nursing school.

...

On one occasion, 9-1-1 had received a call saying that someone had collapsed in one of our parking lots. In our city, we have advanced care paramedics for these types of calls, and normally these guys are right on the ball. This time, however, that was not really the case. They located the patient in the afore-mentioned parking lot and discovered that he was in cardiac arrest. Now, to be clear, this parking lot is literally about fifty meters from our back door. I could have spit on the patient from inside the department, he was that close. Still, the paramedics proceeded to spend forty-five minutes stabilizing the patient before bringing him inside. The ER doctor was livid. He said, "I don't know why they would want to bring him in here. This is just where all the people and machines are." I am fairly certain that he was being sarcastic at the time.

There are always stories on the news about people getting hurt just outside of a hospital. Rather than going out to get the patient, staff will insist that they call an ambulance. These stories always take the tone of how the "mean old hospital staff just left poor granny lying there." To the ordinary eye, it might appear to be a giant waste of resources. Believe it or not, there is method to our madness. First of all, we are not trained to rescue people. The paramedics are. Because we are not trained, we are far more likely to end up getting hurt ourselves. A back injury doesn't only affect us, it affects the entire department and puts every other patient at risk. Not to mention the fact that it can literally ruin a career. It used to be that we were not even covered for such injuries. It was considered outside of our job description. This is no longer the case, but it is still not a practice that we will undertake unless it is absolutely necessary.

With this book, not only do you get so many interesting tidbits. There are also some very valuable public service announcements. Maybe I should be charging more.

Now would perhaps be an ideal time to tell you of *my* back injury. On the day in question, I had a rather large patient who was immobile in bed. She needed her brief changed, so I got one of the care aides to assist me. I am not sure exactly what I did while we were rolling her, but immediately afterwards my entire lower back just seized up. It got so bad that I could no longer stand up straight. I ended up having to go home half an hour later.

By this time, I had gotten rid of my oil-eating car and purchased a new one. It was rather small. I, on the other hand, am not. I spent about half an hour just trying to get into the driver's seat. Every time I tried to get in, I would have to contort myself and pain would go shooting from my back and down my legs. I have no idea how I finally managed to get in. Any tall people out there will understand my struggle.

Now, I am not the kind of person who can just sit around at home. The next day I was back at work, ready to go. For the next two weeks I worked triage (the only job I was really capable of doing with my back out). Meanwhile, the pain just got worse and worse. In the end, my manager had to order me to go home. I was not allowed back until I had been cleared by a doctor.

If you have ever experienced a back injury, then you understand how ironic it can be. To heal, you need to rest. However, if you rest too long in one position, everything gets stiff and it becomes very uncomfortable. You end up having to reposition frequently, which hurts even more. You get up, you lie down. This cycle just repeats itself, over and over again. Back pain is the "Simon Says" of injuries.

This was my first experience with NATH, and I have to say they got my claim going very quickly. I suspect that this is more for their benefit than mine. They had me in rehab right away. I had to go and exercise three times a week. In just over a month I was feeling much improved.

Whenever a nurse is injured on the job, we go through what is called a graduated return-to-work plan (GRTW). This means shorter shifts with a lighter load over a period of several weeks. The load goes up a little each set (a set is four shifts in a row), until the nurse is working full twelve-hour shifts again.

During my GRTW, I noticed that my back was still giving me some difficulty. On one shift, I tweaked it again, and I was in a lot of pain. This is where the rules get a little bit weird. When I raised the question of whether I might require a little more time to get back to 100 percent, I was told that the recovery time for a back injury was six weeks. Therefore, according to their official timetable, I was completely cured. Lucky me. My back still hurts to this day. Perhaps if they had told me of this timetable beforehand, I would have been more eager to comply with their wishes.

Mind you, I must admit that a lower back injury is not as bad as I thought. As I said, the most frustrating thing about a lower back injury is that you never feel comfortable.

It's all just a matter of perspective in the end. Comparatively, if you are going to injure your back at all, then a lower back injury is the way to go. Trust me on this. A few years later, I was working in the streaming area. All our patient charts are kept on clipboards, and after a while (as patients get discharged) we start to gather a collection of empty ones. On this particular day, I had gathered some of these up to bring back to the triage desk. I was trying to carry too many at once and dropped them. For some odd reason, I decided that I could somehow catch them all in midair, like an insane juggler with superpowers. Bad idea. As my hands scrambled madly at empty air, I twisted something in my upper back, right between the shoulder blades. I discovered a whole other level of pain in that moment. It was like a spear going right through my back and out through my chest. I couldn't move, I couldn't even breath. I had to be carried into one of the exam rooms by some paramedics.

Fortunately, this was the last shift of my set. I spent the next four days at home on the couch and it healed up enough that I didn't have to miss any work. Still, I would not wish an upper back injury on anyone. Well, maybe on a *few* people.

This wasn't even the stupidest injury I have ever had. That title goes to a needle-stick injury I suffered on another shift. I had a patient with dementia who was unable to follow directions. She needed to have some blood work drawn. The patient could not understand what was happening and she kept trying to pull away, so the lab technician called me in to hold the patient's arm still. The lab tech stuck the needle in, and the patient decided to yank her arm away from us. Well, that needle flew straight up into the air and fell point down, straight into my thumb. You could not have repeated this sequence of events in a million years.

The chances of actually catching anything from a needle poke are about one-in-three hundred, despite what people think. The chances of contracting hepatitis B are much higher (as high as 30 percent), but all nurses have to be immunized for hep B, at least where I live. I'm also pretty sure that the elderly patient with dementia had not been engaging in many risky activities. Still, there is an extensive procedure that we have to go through each time a needle-stick injury happens. We have to get blood work done at the time and then follow up tests a few months later. It also has to be reported to the hospital, to our manager, and to NATH.

I am lucky. I have had only a few in my career.

This brings to mind another incident. It was particularly scary, though it didn't happen to me. We were in the trauma bay with a patient who had gone into cardiac arrest. There was nothing we could do, so we stopped trying to revive her almost as soon as she arrived. Unfortunately, the doctor caught his finger on a piece of jagged bone that was sticking out of the patient. An injury such as that must be treated the same as a needle poke, for obvious reasons.

As I am sure you can imagine, there is a very short window of time that blood samples can be collected from patients who have died. Without the heart to pump the blood around, gravity tends to take over. As a result, blood will quickly begin to pool toward the patient's back. Knowing this, I immediately got on the phone and called the lab. I told them I needed someone to come right away. It still took a good ten minutes for someone to appear, so we were already getting close to the end of that window. The lab tech proceeded with her blood draw like she would on any other patient. This involved taking time to get all set up, which caused further delay. It was when she started to tie a tourniquet around the patient's arm that I finally lost my patience. A tourniquet works because it creates back pressure in the blood vessels. To do this, there must be forward pressure. In other words, there must be a pulse present. Do you see the problem? I was kind of snippy when I told her to just get on with it. Of course, all that messing around had taken too long and there was no longer any blood that could be drawn. The doctor had to draw the needed sample himself using a special syringe.

The above story illustrates one of the principles I have held onto throughout my practice. In the health care field, we have a great many rules to follow, and no one ever really stops to consider why. I have always believed that we should know the reasons why we do things a certain way, rather than just memorizing the rules. Then, we are far more likely to develop critical thinking skills. This, in turn, allows us to reason out when the rules may not apply. We shouldn't just rely on habits to tell us what to do, because then errors can occur as soon as the usual parameters are no longer present. Use a tourniquet on a live patient, absolutely. On a deceased one, not so much. To be clear, I don't blame the lab technician for any of this. No one had ever taught her anything different.

...

One thing that I imagine will shock a lot of readers is just how much violence nurses face on the job. In fact, nurses are more likely to face violence at work than police officers are. I do not know a single nurse that has not been physically assaulted at some time. This doesn't even include all the verbal abuse we get daily or all the bed pans that get thrown at our heads. I would be hard-pressed to think of a single shift I have worked where I did not have a patient swear at me at least once.

One particular incident involved an inebriated patient who was trying to leave. One of the nurses was attempting to convince her not to go, and I could see that things were escalating quickly. I was standing directly behind the patient when she drew back her fist intending to punch the nurse in the face. I managed to get my arm wrapped around hers, with my hand behind her head. This is a leverage point that can be used to subdue a person (they never taught me *that* in nursing school). By putting pressure on the back of the head, you can force the person forward and down, so that they end up on the floor. Unfortunately, at this point all the other staff members jumped in to help. They were all in front of her, so they enthusiastically grabbed hold of her arms and shoulders. This meant that I could no longer move the patient in a forward direction, the exact thing I was trying to do. We stood there in perfect equilibrium for about thirty seconds, with me pushing one way and them pushing the opposite way. Finally, I looked at everyone and told them to back away.

It's always upsetting when an elderly patient with dementia comes at us, because we don't really know what to do in those cases. I hate trying to physically subdue an older patient because I don't want to break them. They can be so fragile. Besides, there is no worse feeling in the world than the one you get after having to beat up on the elderly. I remember one guy who was probably alive when Stonehenge was first built. He punched me in the shoulder several times, and I felt bad because he was trying so hard to hurt me, but it just wasn't working. It felt more like a tap, to be honest. I think that he would have broken his hand before even raising a bruise on me.

I might be making light of it here, but that level of violence is no laughing matter. It is a constant concern for us. At my hospital, we have a permanent security guard posted in the department during the day. There are panic buttons located everywhere that we can use, if needed. The staff are all trained in violence prevention techniques. These are just a few indications of how seriously we take this issue.

We have long needed a glass barrier at the triage desk. Even in the old department, our requests for such a barrier were denied many times. Apparently, it is felt that this sends an unfriendly message to our patients, as though we don't trust them. Personally, I think seeing my broken and battered body behind the desk would not be a friendly message either. Management still refuses to provide one.

Another handy security measure would be a door between the main lobby and the rest of the department. At this time, there is an open hallway so anyone can walk right in. Again, we don't want to appear unfriendly. Without some type of door, we have no way of controlling who comes in or goes out. This can be especially problematic. We often get patients who are victims of sexual assault or domestic abuse. When we are unsure if the assailant is in police custody, we have to be concerned in case they show up in the ER to finish the job. We have no way of identifying them. We also have no way to stop them from entering. I experienced such an incident several years ago, when the abusive partner showed up and asked to see his girlfriend. This issue becomes even more complicated when dealing with elder abuse, because the entire family will often show up to see the patient. As they all come in together, we cannot single out the individual responsible because we don't have time to stop them as they arrive.

I vividly remember one incident when a patient approached the department carrying a large pipe. I could hear him whacking it on things as he came up the driveway. By the time he entered, he had ditched it somewhere. He denied having it, of course, but the sound of metal hitting metal is very distinctive. Lucky thing he didn't bring it inside. If he had, there was nowhere for us to hide.

After I stopped working there, there was an even more dangerous incident. A man entered the department, jumped over the triage desk, and assaulted one of the nurses. He then proceeded into the back, where he assaulted a patient who had just come in by ambulance. While there, he grabbed a bottle and attacked the second triage nurse. He was chased out the back door by the charge nurse, and he ran off. It turns out that he had a long history of violence. Luckily, there were no serious injuries. Everyone was pretty shaken up, however.

During my time there, we had two separate incidents where someone had threatened to bring a gun to the hospital and start shooting the staff. Again, lucky for us, nothing ever came of these threats.

A few chapters back, I mentioned one of my biggest pet peeves. I get really annoyed at people who stand right behind a patient that I am trying to triage. At one point, I made up a big sign, asking people to please stay back from the desk to give people their privacy. The sign sat on top of a big metal post. This idea worked really well, and for a while we had no more privacy issues. That is, until someone decided to pick up the big metal sign and start swinging it around.

Yeah, we don't need any barriers.

...

My schedule followed one of our regular charge nurse's exactly. I really enjoyed that because she was a lot of fun to work with. When I had first started, she would always try and force me out of my comfort zone. She would just throw me into the deep end of the pool and expect me to swim. For instance, I was nervous about working in the acute room in the old department. Her answer to that was, "You'll be fine. I put you in there tomorrow night." I make it sound like she was a hard ass, but this was actually a good thing. For starters, it made me push myself. Also, she always treated the harder assignments in such a casual manner that I was able to relax about them. Nothing seemed like a big deal to her, which always made me think, "I got this."

She was also one of the bluntest people I have ever met. There was never any mystery about where you stood with her. I remember once hearing the story of a patient who called her a cunt. Without missing a beat, she replied, "That's Mrs. Cunt to you!"

There was one thing, however, that I always hated about working with her. She had this unwavering talent for bringing in the worst possible patients fifteen minutes before shift change. It was like a gift, or perhaps a curse. This was always a lot of fun, especially at the end of a night shift. We would all be watching the clock, willing the hands to move faster so that we could go home to bed. Right at that moment, in would come some guy who was having a big jammer or some mangled motorcycle rider who had wiped out. Whatever it was, you can be assured that most of us were very sleepy at that point. Often, we were only one step away from drooling on ourselves. Suddenly, we would have to pull ourselves together and deal with whatever disaster had just come in the door. We were extremely lucky that we never made any serious mistakes, because none of us were at our best at 7:15 a.m.

...

I did take on two more fourth-year students during this time. They were both smart and very easy to work with, each in their own way.

There was one whom I really enjoyed having as a student. That is because our personalities were very similar. She tended to be quiet and reflective, just like I was.

I do try and keep a professional distance with my students. We are not really there to be friends. I am there to guide them, but also to evaluate them and their work. To do this, I need objectivity, which can be hampered by any friendly feelings that I might have. However, sometimes that distance can make things more awkward. For instance, one day my student and I went on a transfer together. If a patient has to go to another hospital, I always try to take my student with me. It gives them a unique opportunity. On the way back to our hospital, she received a call that her daughter was very sick. For the rest of the trip, we sat in uncomfortable silence. We couldn't even make eye contact. I had no idea what to say to her at that point. I didn't know what was going on with her daughter, and I didn't want to pry. When we got back to the department, she actually tried to go back to work. I had to insist that she go home to be with her family.

After she was finished, we did become very close friends. She was going through a very rough time, and I tried my best to help her get through it. We would sometimes talk for hours, so at least there were no more awkward silences.

The next student that I had was also very good. However, unlike with my previous student, we could not have been more different. She was quite a bit younger than me. I am sure that the entire time we were working together, patients were probably thinking that it was "bring your kid to work day." She was also probably the politest person that I have ever met. She didn't even swear, ever! I usually swear a great deal, so watching my mouth became a full-time job.

Once, we had a patient who was named after a very famous old movie star. I talked with him about it (the patient, not the movie star). As it turned out, his parents had picked that name specifically. Apparently, they were big fans. Afterwards, I told my student that the patient had been named after this actor. "Who?" she said, looking very puzzled. I have never felt so old in my entire life.

I think that if my students had one complaint about me, it would be my endless questions. As I have said, I take great stock in making sure they not only know what to do, but why to do it. I really like to stretch their critical thinking skills, and I expect them to delve deeper in their understanding of what we do. Still, quizzing them at four in the morning is probably a little cruel, and maybe not the surest way to secure their love and admiration. I should probably feel just a little bit sorry for them, but I don't.

Only people who have been preceptors will fully understand just how much work it is. It probably looks so easy to outsiders. After all, the students do most of the heavy lifting. However, those are still my patients. I am still the one who is responsible for their well-being. Because of this, I have to be fully aware of what is going on with them at all times. I also have to maintain the illusion that my student is independent. Otherwise they don't learn anything. It gives them more confidence when they don't have their preceptors looking over their shoulders every five minutes. No one likes being checked up on constantly. As a result, I still have to follow them around all the time. I just can't *appear* to be following them, if you know what I mean. This results in a great deal of sneaking around and surreptitiously listening in on their conversations. In essence, a preceptor must also become a master spy. It is damn well exhausting.

Still, it is so worth it, especially when you get to work with them as colleagues later on. Remember the student I had who tried to start the IV in the wrong direction? A few years later, she had a patient that none of us will ever forget. I believe we had not been in the new department very long. Perhaps a year or so at most. A patient was brought in by ambulance, and she seemed absolutely determined to die. We had to stop and resuscitate her while getting her from the ambulance to the trauma bay. This continued on for hours, until we shipped her out. This was perhaps one of the hardest events that I have ever witnessed, but my former student handled every minute of it with poise and professionalism. I have rarely felt so proud.

Another job that I performed frequently was orienting new employees. Sometimes, these nurses were brand new to the ER. Sometimes, they had a great deal of experience, but were new to our department. Either way, I was there to show them the ropes. I had to make sure that they knew the proper procedures, that they could find everything, and that they knew who to call when they needed something. I would also spend some time going over which doctors are better to approach, and which ones to avoid. All our doctors are great, but a few can be a little gruff if you are pestering them for something like an order for pain medication. This is especially true when a nurse is new, because the doctors don't know him or her yet. Orientations are usually a lot more relaxed, because I'm not really teaching them anything. Just the odd trick or two that I have picked up over the years. Most of the time, I simply allow them to direct me, to tell me what they want me to do. Then I just answer any questions they might have. Sometimes, I just have to sit on my ass and watch them go. Good times.

...

Without a doubt, the worst day we ever had in our emergency department involved a workplace shooting with multiple casualties. I always hear about such events on the news, but it is always something that occurs "somewhere else." Not in our little town (not so little anymore, I suppose). I was just finishing my night shift, but I volunteered to stay for a few extra hours. I knew that every single nurse would be busy dealing with the casualties that were coming in, so an extra pair of hands would be very useful. Even hands as tired as mine were.

I figured that I could best serve the department by manning the triage desk. This also seemed like the safest place for me to be, considering I had already worked a full twelve hours. One thing about having worked in the ER for a long time is that I have become pretty confident in my abilities. This confidence allowed me to deflect many would-be patients coming in with simpler complaints. I stayed at the triage desk for the next three hours, and I must have sent half the people away.

"You have a urinary tract infection? Right now, I can guarantee that you will not be seen for many hours. It would be a much better idea to go to a clinic or to your family doctor."

That can be a risky tactic sometimes. I do make mistakes, just like anyone else. If someone goes home and dies, I would be in a great deal of trouble. Still, when you have that many critical patients rolling in at once, the reality is that any lower level patients are going to end up *way* down on the priority list. Even after we deal with the all the critical patients, which will take many hours, we still have to see all the other patients in the department who were already waiting when they arrived.

Once I explained what was happening, none of the patients I told to go away tried to argue with me. Most were happy to be on their way because it was quite obvious how awful things were at that point. There was literally a trail of blood from the ambulance bay to the trauma room. Outside, there were ambulances everywhere. There were paramedics, police officers, and firefighters all over the place. Everyone had a look of shocked disbelief on their faces. We also had security everywhere because, at first, no one was sure if the shooter had been accounted for. There was genuine concern that he might just show up. The entire department was in complete chaos.

One thing about living in a smaller city is that many of the people are connected somehow. As a transplant, I didn't know anyone, but several of the other staff members did. One of our nurses had a relative who worked at the office where the shooting had occurred. For those staff members, there was a great deal of fear and uncertainty as well. Details were very sketchy at first, so people were often left to speculate about their loved ones. For many, there was nothing they could do but worry. It is amazing to me just how professional the team I work with can be when the chips are down. Not one single person blinked. Even as they fretted over friends and family members, every single nurse and doctor there (and others) performed with the utmost diligence. That is something that we can all be extremely proud of.

As an example, one of the paramedics was just sitting behind the triage desk, crying. The patient that she had brought in was a friend of hers. The strength of character that it takes to do something like that is beyond belief. Having to then go out again, to continue to do your job, that is absolutely legendary.

I really didn't want to end the chapter on such a depressing note. Luckily, I remembered another story. You might recall that my entire reason for getting into nursing in the first place was based on an episode of *ER*. Well, I ended up in precisely the same situation. I had a patient who was also dying. There was absolutely nothing we could do for him. He was still fully conscious, so he was well aware that he was going to die soon. I just sat with him and talked for hours. Unlike the show, I wasn't there when he did die, but I hope that I eased his passing just a little bit.

This illustrates why all ER nurses are going to hell. It was a case that involved something that none of us had ever heard of before. It was so out of the ordinary that we actually had to look it up. The process his body was going through was very complex and very fascinating. It was really horrible for the patient, but for me it was all so very interesting.

HAVE YOU TRIED UNPLUGGING
IT AND PLUGGING IT BACK IN?

I t was around four years ago that things started to go very wrong in the emergency department. By this point, I had been working as an ER nurse for ten years. At that time, the powers that be had decided to introduce a new computer program, and our hospital was "volunteered" to be the test site. If you are reading this and do not work in health care, you might be tempted to skip ahead, but I am hoping that you won't. This chapter is a little bit technical, yes. However, the reason I have included this story is because it will provide further insight into my own frame of mind, especially since these events contributed a great deal to my current state of mental health. Besides, the sheer irony of the entire situation should be very entertaining when seen from the outside. Even if you do not understand the more technical aspects, I think that it will still be good for a laugh or two.

As I was saying, we suddenly found ourselves having to contend with a new computer program. The whole purpose of this new program was to provide an integrated platform for charting on our patients. There were four main objectives.

The first was to organize the charts in a more concise way. In paper charts, information ends up all over the place, as everyone has their own unique way of doing things. It can be difficult to retrieve that information later on. This makes it almost impossible to create an accurate picture of a patient's progress, especially from a linear perspective. By providing standardized charting forms, all information would be located where it was supposed to be. Therefore, such information would be easy to find and track. Also, most of the charting would be streamlined into boxes that could simply be ticked off if they applied. This was meant to make charting faster. It was also intended to avoid charting that might be extraneous and unnecessary. Some nurses can fill pages and pages of irrelevant information in a chart.

Second, it was to provide a charting platform that would follow the patient around wherever they went. The idea was to get every health care professional on board. In this way, the chart would always be available for any professional who needed access to it. Family doctors, other hospitals, clinics, etc. Everyone would instantly be able to see what everyone else had done over the entire course of the patient's life, or at least as far back as the electronic chart went. It also provided a platform for all the different disciplines to chart in. Nurses would have access to notes from physiotherapy. Doctors could see what the pharmacist had written.

Third, the program would be able to tabulate and display statistics for each site (hospital, clinic, etc.), as well as across sites. Modern health care runs on numbers. It's not enough, in this day and age, to do our jobs. We are beholden to the taxpayers, and we must be able to *prove* that we are doing our jobs. In other words, we have to be able to provide data in order to justify our expenditures. Stats also aid us in directing resources more efficiently. If we can see that a particular site has experienced a sudden spike in the number of patients they see, then that site can take those numbers and use them to justify hiring additional staff.

Fourth, it was meant to ensure that safety standards were being strictly adhered to when administering medications. The whole idea was to eliminate errors. Every patient was given a scannable wristband to wear upon admission. Each medication was also scannable. We were required to scan the patient and then the medication, and the two had to match up. This was done in order to verify that the right medication was being given to the right patient at the right time. If any of the information was incorrect, such as a medication being given too early, the computer program would alert the nurse responsible. It also was designed to flag high risk medications (such as blood thinners) so that the nurse could take extra precautions.

This, of course, was all in theory. The reality was very different.

It all began with one of the most insane decisions ever undertaken by a medical institution. The project was quite extensive, given the goals that I have outlined above. As a result, it had been subject to endless delays and cost overruns. There was enormous pressure to get the whole project online quickly. Also, the budgetary year was about to end. For these reasons, the project was rushed out way before it was ready, and several fundamental steps had been skipped over entirely during development.

For starters, all new computer programs go through what is called a beta test. This is when the developers and programmers introduce the software to the people who will actually be using it. This is all done in a simulated setting, allowing users to see how the program functions in real life situations, but without real life consequences. The whole purpose is to ensure that the program performs up to expectations and to correct any program glitches that may pop up. This step was never done, or at least this is my understanding.

Also skipped was any attempt to collaborate with staff when designing the interface. This was particularly evident in the medication portion of the program. It was designed by a pharmacist, with no thought about how it would be used by doctors and nurses in an actual clinical setting.

Next, training of the staff was both inadequate and incomplete. The nurses were provided with only two days of training. The physicians got even less. Our entire work environment was about to change, and we were essentially going in blind.

At this point, I must clarify that I am a huge fan of electronic charting. I firmly believe that our profession needs to embrace every technological tool at our disposal, especially when it enhances the care that we are able to provide. Of course, being able to view a patient's entire history will result in fewer mistakes. It also lessens overlap of care (people doing the same things) and increases continuity. It is an idea that's time has come.

Unfortunately, that is definitely *not* what happened here. We paid for a Cadillac, but we ended up with a '77 Pinto instead.

To begin with, the entire program suffered from design flaws, right from the beginning. It was clunky, slow, and counterintuitive to use.

Let's begin by using this very book as an example. I am writing this at home (and in various coffee shops around town) using Word. Many of you are probably very familiar with Word. I have never taken a course in how to use Word, nor have I had to consult with anyone. That is because the entire program is designed for ease of use. Everything I need to find on the interface is somewhere that is easy to locate. Things flow logically because every function I need to use is in a location that makes sense. It's all right where it is supposed to be, making Word extremely user-friendly. Even when I am not sure how to do something, the answer is readily accessible. (Hey Microsoft, I am expecting some form of kickback for that little blurb, just so you are aware.)

Our new program had none of these features. Everything was overcomplicated. Nothing flowed. None of the tools seemed to be arranged in any logical order. Even the forms themselves were not organized in a manner that would make sense for us, the people who were supposed to be using them. This wasn't the fault of the company that designed the software either. It was *our* programmers who had designed all this.

For example, let's start with something small: the triage screen. Now, keep in mind that these mistakes could easily have been avoided simply by consulting with someone who has actually worked triage before. Instead, it was left to the computer programmers. Because of this, the spot where we were supposed to fill in vital signs for patients when they arrived was in the opposite order to how it was arranged on the ambulance forms. This meant that we had to train our paramedics to read their vitals backwards to us, from right to left. Now, this may seem like a very minor problem. It only took a few seconds at most, but what's a few seconds times two hundred people a day?

Listing patient allergies was an even more complicated process. We would have to start by clicking on the button for allergies on the triage screen. This would bring up a second screen that listed any known allergies for the patient. If there was a new allergy to add in, we had to click on the button saying "add new allergy." This brought up a third screen. We would then have to search for the appropriate allergy and highlight it. Then, we would be taken back to the second screen. Here we would have to plug in what type of allergy it was (medication, environmental, or food), as well as the patient's reaction to said allergen. Next, we had to click on the button that said confirm, so that the new allergy was locked into the patient's chart. This would take us back to the triage screen. We had to do this with each new allergy. Just imagine what this was like with a patient with multiple allergies to chart coming into the ER for the first time.

Once the patient made it past the triage desk, things did not get any better. For the primary nurse, the patient assessment forms were just as bad. The tick boxes were way too extensive. Yet, somehow, they also managed to be incomplete. I am not even sure how they accomplished that. Items that we used on a regular basis were missing, replaced by options that made absolutely no sense. For instance, under chief complaint I could chart anthrax exposure, but not other far more common complaints. In fourteen years, I have yet to see an anthrax exposure.

Also, when an accurate option was not available in the tick boxes, it would have been helpful if we were able to write it in. However, no place had been provided for us to input any free text. When such a place was introduced a few months later (after many complaints from staff), it was still very limited in scope. We had one little box we could write in, and we only had a limited number of characters.

Even starting an IV became a chore, because I would have to chart where the IV had been placed. The simplest thing would have been to list the most common sites first, such as left arm, right arm, etc. Instead, we got a lengthy and randomized list. We would have to scroll through multiple possibilities until we found the right location. Some of the areas listed were feet, scalp, upper thigh, etc. None of these are areas we access for IVs very often, if ever.

The entire program was so unnecessarily complicated that, for the first couple of months, all the nurses were chained to the computers constantly. We no longer had any time to spend with the patients. Instead of exerting our efforts doing actual nurse stuff, we had to spend endless hours slogging through the forms just so that we could chart. The great irony is that we now had less to chart because we were no longer able to see as many people. The entire department came to a grinding halt. Wait times tripled. The patients were also getting fed up. All they saw were nurses with their eyes glued to the computer monitors, so the patients just assumed that we were deliberately ignoring them. Tempers began to flare.

To be clear, not everything was negative. One positive function of the program was the ease with which we could now order most tests. By opening the screens for lab and X-ray, we could instantly send requests to the appropriate people. Moments later, those people would appear with all their equipment in hand. In the old days, we would have to phone each person, and half the time they wouldn't be able to answer right away. Now we just clicked and all the lab tests we needed would print up right next to the lab station.

With the program, we could also pull vitals right from the bedside monitors and place them appropriately in the chart. We could do this with a single click of the mouse. That was a great improvement from the past, when we would have had to write them in ourselves, one by one.

Even this relatively simple procedure had a few glitches, however. Urine samples were a big problem. Unlike blood work, the nurses were responsible for collecting all urine samples (I like to joke that the hospital is the only place where you can hand people a jar of pee, and they will say thank you). If the nurses ordered a urine sample, a label would print up for us. The location it would print up, however, seemed totally randomized. There were often several nurses aimlessly wandering the halls looking for lost urine labels. Then, if we never managed to locate said label, printing up a repeat label was next to impossible.

The most infuriating part of the entire process was that the administrators knew what would happen well ahead of time. We were not the first institution to use a program such as this. In other hospitals, workload would increase by 25 percent in the first few months after implementation. Every single time. It would have made sense, then, to increase staffing levels by 25 percent to compensate. That would be the logical move. Unfortunately, it seemed that there was no money left to bring extra people in. The remaining staff were, of course, unable to keep up with the increased amount of work. We had to just continue on our own.

Without a doubt, the most cumbersome component of the program was the medication section. In fact, it was a complete nightmare to use at first. Scanning medications was an extremely slow process, which does not fly in an emergency room. I think we scanned the medications for about a week until one of our more enterprising nurses found a loophole that we could use. By clicking on the screen in a certain way, we could bypass the scanning altogether. All that happened was a red box would pop up, saying, "are you sure you don't want to scan?" Why, yes I am! I would be very surprised if anyone in our department ever scanned a medication again.

There was a whole list of other complaints because of the pharmacy piece as well. A good example would be when we would receive an order for antibiotics. Now, being an emergency department, not all our medications are given on a schedule. When a patient is admitted, often we would get an order that said something like, "Antibiotic three times a day, and give an initial dose now." Well, the computer would automatically assign scheduled doses for three different times throughout the day, and they would be at very specific times (say 9 a.m., 3 p.m., and 9 p.m.). If the initial dose was too close to the first of the scheduled times (such as 12:30 a.m.), the nurses would simply have altered the other doses a little so that they could all be accommodated, without any of the doses being too close together (initial dose at 12:30 a.m., then doses at noon, 4 p.m. and 10 p.m.). Hopefully, that makes sense to you. We call it staggering. The computer was unable to improvise like this, however. Often, we wouldn't be able to input the initial dose at all because it was too close in time to the first scheduled dose. The computer would just flash angry messages on the screen and beep repeatedly, like a car alarm going off.

Another problem with the pharmacy section was that we were sometimes given orders for medications with variable doses. The dose could be altered according to certain pre-set parameters. A good example of this would be a diabetic on an insulin infusion. The doctor's order would say, "If the patient's blood sugar is this, reduce the dose to this." The computer didn't understand that at all. It took several months to correct this.

The funniest part was that the program would record each of these instances as prevented medication errors. The pharmacists would then use these statistics to justify how useful the program was. "Look, I know it's hard, but we caught one thousand medication errors last month. That proves it's much safer." Of course, they didn't realize that the system was creating many of these errors in the first place. It's like if I went into a store and stole a bunch of stuff. Then I go to the front counter, admit my crime, and turn myself in. Afterwards, I give myself a jolly old pat on the back for catching the thief red-handed. Of course, that sounds ridiculous. Yet, that is exactly what the program was doing.

For the doctors, the whole process was even more cumbersome. Instead of just writing down orders, which is what they used to do, they now had to type them in on the computer. This process was extremely long and arduous. A complicated patient could take hours to enter. Errors in dosages happened frequently because the lists they had to choose from were unclear and overly long. For the hospital doctors, who might have thirty patients a day to see, the entire process became impossible to complete within the time they were supposed to be on shift. I would frequently see the doctors still typing away, sixteen hours into a shift. Needless to say, their expressions were not happy while doing this.

Up until this time, processing orders had been the duty of the unit clerks. In fact, it was their primary function. Now, that duty had been taken away from them and reassigned to the physicians. All of a sudden, the unit clerks found themselves with very little to do all day. They had the time to enter the orders, and they had the necessary training. However, for some unfathomable reason, it was decided that the already overwhelmed doctors would have to do this themselves from now on. The unit clerks did eventually take over other duties, but for those first few weeks they spent a great deal of time fighting boredom.

I understand the *intention* behind all these changes. The purpose was to slow the whole process down and to make the doctors more accountable for their orders. This was all supposed to reduce errors. However, the realities of our work environment should have been taken into account at some point. As I said earlier, you can't increase the amount of work a person is expected to do without also providing more people to do that work. You can't tell people to speed up and slow down at the same time. It's simply not possible.

There were also the times when the program just didn't work, where random errors would occur for no apparent reason. Every program contains such errors. Usually, most are discovered and corrected before implementation. This is why software is supposed to be rigorously tested prior to use. Not in our case, apparently. One night, when I was in charge, the computer started to assign random numbers to patients. Every patient in the system has a number that stays with them forever. This is called the medical record number (MRN). It is never supposed to change because this is how we know that you are you. It is also how we gain access to your medical history. Well, for some reason, the computer started assigning brand new MRNs to patients that we had seen in the past. This was a serious problem, as it meant that we could not access old charts for any of these individuals. The situation became critical when an error very nearly resulted in the death of one patient.

When I called up the IT desk, I was told that because it was a weekend, no help would be available to us until the following Monday.

Me: "Isn't there some sort of emergency protocol?"

IT guy: "Yes."

Me: "Well, you need to implement it."

IT guy: "I can't. No one has told me what it is."

Me: "Seriously, no one has told you what to do in a case like this?"

IT guy: "No."

Me: "Well, do you have a supervisor?"

IT guy: "Yes, he'll be in on Monday."

By the end of this conversation, any sense of reason that I had previously possessed had deserted me. Instead, I was just yelling into the phone. I told him that I didn't care who he had to wake up, I wanted the problem fixed that night. I wasn't going to wait around while lives were at risk. This is what happens when a system is designed by people who will never use it. For us, this was a critical issue that needed an immediate response. For them, it was just a random glitch that could be fixed at their earliest convenience.

None of these problems would have been insurmountable if they could have been corrected easily. Unfortunately, no one had thought to make the program modular. Given the complexity of the system we were using, this had a major impact on how quickly the computer programmers were able to correct problems. For example, they couldn't just pull out the pharmacy part and fix it in one go, because the pharmacy section was connected to all of the other sections. As a result, they had to fix each individual problem as it happened. It took four years to get the program working as well as it should have been right from the start. A modular design would have made this process simpler and faster.

This is but a small sample of the problems we had. There were many, many others. So many, in fact, that there were scores of people who were running around with the sole purpose of helping us when we ran into difficulty. We couldn't afford additional medical staff, but apparently we could afford to pay hordes of tech people!

A few of the more enterprising doctors even had their own personal tech person. Their newfound assistants would follow them around and do all the computer entry tasks. In other words, the program that was designed specifically to make doctors more accountable was so unwieldy to use that it had created the opposite effect. Not to mention that the unit clerks, who are highly trained professionals, had now been supplanted by untrained technicians doing the same job. The entire situation became thick with irony.

Now remember, we had been chosen for this "very special honor." We were the first. Perhaps instituting a brand-new program at one of your busiest hospitals is not such a great plan. Maybe picking a smaller hospital would have been more appropriate. This is especially true when you consider that no effort had been taken to work out any of the problems beforehand.

Of course, It didn't take long before rebellions started. Health care staff are a raucous bunch, and we do not take kindly to those who seek to make our lives more difficult. We have more than enough stress as it is. The physicians held several meetings to discuss the problem, one of which I managed to attend. At each meeting, there was a palpable seething rage. Every single doctor in the hospital seemed to be fed up.

The first to drop out was the ICU. Their physicians simply refused to use the program anymore, and they went back to paper charts. The ER was next, but we were only allowed to go halfway. We would use paper for the ER patients and the computer for admitted ones. The day we went back to paper was the first time I had seen the staff happy in months. Everyone in the entire department looked like it was the middle of Mardi Gras.

The internal medicine doctors tried to do something similar. Unfortunately, there were a few in their number who broke ranks, so their entire rebellion fell apart. Administration then came down hard on the instigators. Some of the internal med doctors chose to leave the hospital completely, which led to total chaos. One was even fined. As a direct result, many shifts could no longer be covered as there were no longer enough doctors to fill them. The ICU doctors found themselves having to work internal medicine shifts in addition to covering their own department, just so the hospital could keep functioning. I swear that some of the ICU doctors just seemed to live at the hospital for weeks on end. There's only so long that such a pace can be sustained without serious consequences for patient care.

The entire culture of the hospital began to change. The managers seemed to become angrier and angrier at the staff. Management appeared unable to distinguish between electronic charting as an idea (which was good) and the reality that we had been presented with (which was very, very bad). As a result, they defended the program vigorously. The company line was that the program was fine, it was just that the staff were all stupid. We weren't paying attention, or we were deliberately being negative. I was told, to my face, that I was the problem on more than one occasion.

Complaints were ignored, and those that persisted in complaining were let go (often on trumped up accusations). Our workplace became like a dictatorship, where people would just disappear mysteriously from one day to the next.

Our working environment quickly graduated from merely strange to downright absurd. For example, in the middle of all of this, someone decided to have a "staff appreciation day." Somehow, free hot dogs were going to make everything better. "Our computer program isn't working because you're all stupid and lazy. Would you like relish with that?" I felt as though I were stuck in some repeating episode of *The Twilight Zone*. As far as I know, hardly anyone attended their little soiree.

In case you are thinking that it might have been us, let me say this: One of our doctors is a programmer. He actually knows how to write code. He couldn't understand it. I watched some of the smartest people I know break down in frustration daily. Not everyone is good with change, I admit. However, when I see the copers not coping, that's when I start to worry. That's when I say to myself, "It's not us. We're not the problem here."

Other hospitals were starting to get wind of this by now. The staff from other sites were now banding together and flat out refusing to have the program implemented where they worked. Suddenly, the main reason for getting the program in the first place—to create an integrated chart for each patient—was no longer valid. We couldn't see what other nurses and doctors were doing with our patients because they wouldn't use the chart we were forced to use. It took two more years before they could force it on another hospital, and that only happened because they built an entirely new facility and installed the program before anyone moved in. No one really had a chance to object.

Whenever we transferred a patient to another hospital, we would end up having to print off the entire chart because, otherwise, the second hospital would not have had access to it.

The atmosphere became so toxic at work that an independent audit had to be ordered. The report found that bullying and harassment were endemic within the facility. Employee morale was nonexistent, and cohesiveness had completely broken down. Everyone was miserable, and a gaping chasm had opened up between the staff and management.

It was obvious by now what a disaster the whole enterprise was shaping up to be. Suddenly, the big boss in our area resigned his position to "spend more time with the family." I'm not saying that he didn't, but the timing seemed very suspicious to me. Many of the people responsible suddenly found themselves reassigned to new jobs. Of course, it was the only woman of the group who got fired. I am told that there may have been additional reasons for this, but, again, it seemed just a little suspicious.

Things did get better. After four years, I can now say that the program is almost workable. Many of the problems have been corrected. It's still not very user-friendly, but now the staff has learned where everything is located within the program anyway. There are parts we still don't know very well, but some clever people in the hospital have been able to figure out work-arounds and passed them along to the rest of us. In other words, we cheat. Many of the other sites still have no immediate plans to implement it.

The hospital has also taken many steps to improve the workplace environment. A new committee was started, and its sole purpose was to improve workplace culture. Staff were asked to provide feedback and ideas. People were actually listened too for a change. Still, it is a slow process, and there is an enormous amount of damage to repair. At least the process has begun.

WHERE DID ALL THESE PEOPLE COME FROM?

I 'm not exactly sure when things first started to get bad for me. Thinking back, it was all rather like the analogy of the frog in the boiling water. Put a frog in a boiling pot and it will immediately jump out. However, if you put the frog in cold water and then gradually heat it up, the frog will just sit there and happily boil to death. I am not sure if this is true, and if it is then frogs must be a special kind of stupid. Still, you get the point. There were no sudden changes to my mental state. The changes were far more subtle than that, and they occurred over a long period of time.

The department had been through so many difficult periods those last few years, and this was especially hard on the senior staff. We felt overworked and undervalued. More importantly, we felt silenced. This period of time saw the second great exodus of people from our department. Every one of my teammates seemed to be leaving at the same time. My support network was rapidly unravelling.

Perhaps the biggest challenge for us was the changing dynamics that occurred within our local community. We are a very busy department, as you already know. What had always been our saving grace each year was that we also had lulls, particularly during the summer months. Usually, once flu and pneumonia season came to an end, our numbers would drop off just a little. This allowed the staff a chance to catch our breath. We were still busy, of course, but not as busy.

That began to change, drastically. Over a period of about two years, our city experienced a very large influx of seniors. One nearby town grew by over five thousand people. This, in turn, created a surge of patients coming to the hospital. As most were older, they often had multiple medical conditions. They would almost always require more complex care. The whole system became overloaded because, once again, no one had thought to make extra resources available.

In the emergency department, this translated into a genuine crisis. Though the actual number of patients we saw in a day stayed about the same, what did change was the type of patients we were seeing. More patients came in that were not mobile. Thus, many required stretchers. Until this time, having patients in the hallway was a rarity. Now, it became the norm. Our normal workload in the monitored area had been three or four patients per nurse. Suddenly, it was not unusual to have six to eight patients per nurse.

The complexity of the care we had to provide also increased. This meant that more patients needed to be admitted to the hospital, as they would have been unable to manage at home. Of course, this creates a rather large problem, because a hospital is a finite space. There are only so many people that can be crammed in at any given time, even when you start stuffing them into TV rooms and broom closets. The hospital was running at 130 percent capacity or above, every single day. Think of it this way: If you try to cram too much toilet paper down the toilet, things are going to back up, making a rather large mess. This is exactly what happened in our department. The floors can only take so many people. Once they were full, we were forced to keep all the rest. The toilet exploded, and we ended up covered in crap.

Remember those nice, private rooms we had? Suddenly, they were not so private anymore. At least two of our larger rooms had to be doubled up, with stretchers side by side. We used these to house inpatients, so that we could free up space for incoming patients. The department had to invest in dividers so that we could provide even a little bit of privacy.

Several times, there would be two patients on oxygen in the same room. The oxygen supply was located on one of the walls. We were able to hook the patient closest to that wall up without any difficulties. The patient on the other side of the room would need to have several oxygen tubes connected together in order to reach it. On a few occasions, I very nearly tripped over these extra-long O2 lines because they often dangled onto the floor.

In conditions such as these, it is next to impossible to provide each patient with the care they deserve. There is the old saying that any landing you can walk away from is a good one. That pretty much sums up how I would feel at the end of my shift each day. Not the pride of a job well done, but the consolation that nothing bad had happened, that no one had died. That is a pretty crappy way to feel every day. As nurses (well, most of us anyway), we take great pride in looking after our patients. It is the only thing that makes the bad days tolerable. Taking that away from us is a recipe for disaster, because it is not sustainable. Nurses are people too, and there is only so much emotional battering that we can take. Eventually, anyone can break if you apply enough pressure. That is exactly what happened to me.

It was the inpatients, I think, that ended up suffering the most. Remember, they are never our priority. Some days, my only contact with them would be checking in every few hours to make sure they were still alive. Other than that, I gave them their medication. That was it. There were days when I seriously could not have picked my admitted patients out of a lineup. What made this situation even worse was that sometimes I would see the same admitted patients throughout my set. That was how long some of them were stuck there.

Some days, even the emergency patients would not receive good care. On the really bad days, it became our routine to stabilize and move on. Patients would always receive our best when they first came in, but after that it was on to the next, and the next, and the next. To put this in perspective, every new patient requires twenty to thirty minutes of our time when they first arrive. That is how long it takes us to assess them, get them hooked up to the monitors, pop an IV in, and so forth. Add on a couple of minutes if they needed something right away, such as a medication. For six patients, that is around three hours, give or take. In that three hours, two of those patients have been discharged home and two new patients have arrived. This means that we are already an hour behind.

What was even more alarming was that we were forced to put regular patients into the trauma room almost every day. Not only does this tie up a staff member, but it also limits our capacity to respond if a real trauma shows up. Those were the days that really fried our nerves, because we knew that there was absolutely nowhere to go.

You must remember that people who work in health care tend to be a little obsessive, especially when it comes to picking at our own shortcomings. Just imagine what happens to our mental state when all we feel is failure. It haunts us. I can clearly recall carrying around this feeling, deep in the pit of my stomach. It felt like a knotted ball that refused to release. Every. Single. Day!

Then the summer came, and the usual lull did not materialize. As you can imagine, this had a profound effect on the staff's morale. There was no time for us to recoup, no chance to recharge our strength. Work became more of a marathon, with each of us struggling to go just one more day. On and on and on.

Night shifts also began to see a rise in patient volumes. There is this funny tendency in human nature. We have an idea, and for some bizarre reason we think that this idea is ours alone. No one else in the history of the universe has ever come up with a plan as brilliant as ours. That is never the case. So many people would decide to come in during the night, assuming that it would be less busy. Well, guess what? Seems that everyone else had the exact same idea. A third of all the patients we saw were coming in on night shifts when I left.

What really made me angry was that these conditions were so easily preventable. All it would have taken was for someone in authority to open a newspaper. That's why I knew what was happening, so why didn't management? "Oh look, boss person. Our population is rising. Most of them are elderly. Perhaps we should include that in our plans for the coming year, don't you think?" Apparently, no one did.

There were days when I considered bringing in my tent from home, just so we would have some more space. After all, we had a large grassy area out front that wasn't being used for anything. Maybe some of the admitted patients could have a campout. Hospital food cooking over an open fire. I even suggested to one of the doctors that he bring his VW van in. That's another two beds right there.

...

The first symptom that I noticed was a migraine that wouldn't go away. Most of the time, it was just a dull ache. However, when it came on full force, it could be crippling in intensity. This started about a year and a half before I left.

Unsurprisingly, this was a little alarming for me, at first. After about a week, I figured I must be having some sort of stroke (all nurses are terrible hypochondriacs). However, strokes don't usually tend to linger on like that, so I was able to relax a little.

On one occasion, the pain was so intense that I had to check myself in as a patient. The doctor who saw me managed to get me in to see a neurologist. He also ordered some blood tests and a CT scan of my brain. Thankfully, all my tests came back normal (yes, they did find a brain in there). The headache still refused to go away though.

It was only about a week or two later that I got in to see the neurologist. He decided that the next step was a spinal tap, in case it was some type of meningitis. I can still remember showing up to the neurologist's office. I was shown into an exam room to wait, and there, next to the exam table, was a tray with the biggest damn needle I had ever laid eyes on. Picture a straw with a pointy end. I just about fainted right there, and I immediately began to plot my escape. Fortunately, I had not quite cemented my plans when the doctor came in. Turned out that the needle was not for me at all. In fact, he had decided against doing a spinal tap entirely. I was so relieved that I just about passed out a second time.

His official diagnosis was lack of sleep brought on by shift work. Apparently, this type of headache is quite common in nurses. Constantly switching back and forth between day and night shifts disrupts the normal sleep patterns, so we never get adequate rest. He told me to start taking melatonin, which did help a little. The headache never went away completely, though.

It always amazes me what the human body can get used to. I have developed a real appreciation for those with chronic conditions, as I now had an intimate understanding of what they go through every day. When a person has constant pain, there comes a point at which it starts to seem normal. It's as if I had forgotten what it was like to not have that pain. As time wore on, there were days I would not even notice it was there, unless I actually thought about it. Then, of course, there were quite a few days that the pain would make its presence felt. "Hey, you've been ignoring me. That hurts my feelings, so now you will pay." Increased stress was always the trigger. On those days, it was like having a pickax driven through the side of my head and into my brain (or, at least, what I imagine that would feel like). I also became a regular patient in my own department.

During this time, I did happen upon one positive aspect of our new computer system. There was a clinic right by my house that was also using the program. I had to go there on one occasion, as the headache was bad that day. When the doctor came in, I don't think that he realized who I was. Not knowing that I was an ER nurse, or that I was friends with the first doctor I had seen, he essentially repeated verbatim what the first doctor had said. It was obvious that he had read what was on my chart and simply repeated it, word for word. So, if I did have to say something nice about the program, it is that doctors who aren't sure what they are talking about can now sound smart.

About four months later, a new symptom began to manifest itself. It only happened a few times, but, on each occasion, it would freak the hell out of me. The first time, I was returning from the cafeteria with my lunch. I was on my way back to the staff room to eat, taking a route I have taken over a thousand times. Suddenly, I had this feeling that I didn't know where I was. It was as if everything was suddenly unrecognizable to me. I knew that I should know, but I didn't. The only way to describe the sensation is that it was almost dreamlike, like everything was just a little off. "Ok, now this *must* be a stroke." It lasted only a few seconds, and then everything returned to normal. This required more tests, but again there was nothing to find. There were a few more events like this over the next year, and I just figured that they were related to the headaches somehow. It was only much later that I learned the real cause. I was reading a book and it described the feeling exactly. Apparently, what I had been experiencing were called dissociative episodes.

The worst thing about stress related symptoms is that they can become a vicious circle. The more symptoms you have, the more stressed you feel, and so on.

As time progressed, several more symptoms began to present themselves. I became more and more irritable. This continued to progress to the point that I would experience genuine rage at the slightest provocation, especially at work. I can recall several instances when I would be triaging a patient for some minor complaint, and I would literally have to fight the urge to reach across the desk and punch them in the face. Given the environment I was working in, where there are so many aggravating factors, it became quite problematic to have such a short fuse.

Once, a patient's husband came up to the triage desk and complained about how long his wife had been waiting. He was very angry and belligerent, with his voice raised. He even leaned over my desk a few times in an aggressive manner. Now, this type of behavior is simply unacceptable. Still, I am a professional and I am supposed to act like one. My role is to try and diffuse the situation, not to make it worse. Instead, I completely lost my temper. He was getting in my face, so I stood up and got right in his. The two of us faced off across the desk for several minutes, just yelling at one another. I am sure that a few people probably came in through the front door, turned around, and went right back out again upon seeing this exchange.

My co-workers were not immune to my wrath either. There was one episode where a new patient was brought in to one of our isolation rooms. It wasn't my section, but the nurse for that area was fairly new, and she was feeling a little overwhelmed. The triage nurse asked me if I could go in to do the assessment on this patient. I was not thrilled by this idea, as I already had eight patients of my own. In addition, the new patient had something (I can't remember exactly what) that required full isolation precautions. This meant that I would have to spend even more time getting all the protection gear on and off. Still, the patient was quite short of breath and needed attention quickly, so off I went. I emerged about twenty minutes later, having finished my assessment. I had also given the patient something to make her breathing easier. That's when I noticed that someone was in with one of *my* patients. Curious as to what was going on, I poked my head in to the room. The triage nurse and one of our care aides was busy cleaning and changing the patient in bed. I asked what they were doing, and the triage nurse said, "Apparently, we're doing your job." Now, I knew that she was just kidding around, but that was the wrong time to be snarky. My temper flared like a bomb going off. I yelled at them both, then walked out of the room and slammed the door shut behind me. This was all done right in front of the patient, which is also completely unprofessional. The triage nurse is one of my very favorite people, and I don't think that I have ever even apologized to her for this incident. I must remember to do so.

You are probably thinking, "What a jerk!" right about now. If it improves your opinion of me at all, I would like to point out that she lost her temper with me only a few weeks later. This doesn't justify what I did, but it does assuage my guilt just a little bit. I think that we were all under so much pressure.

At home, I noticed that the opposite reaction was happening. It's almost as if my brain was trying to compensate for my angry outbursts at work. Instead of rage, I just felt really sad and weepy all the time. A sappy commercial would come on TV, and I would feel like bawling my eyes out. Little setbacks would send me into a depression. It was as if every emotional response became exaggerated and overwhelming.

My energy level at home became nonexistent. I stopped doing almost everything, even things that I had previously enjoyed. At that time, I was an avid online gamer. Nothing can make the stress melt away like coming home after work and killing a bunch of people (in the game, I mean). Suddenly, it was as if I just couldn't be bothered anymore. I even cancelled my subscription for the game and gave up playing altogether. Instead, I would just lie in bed and watch TV until it was time to go to sleep every night.

I also used to read a great deal, but I lost interest in that as well. I doubt that I even picked up a book for an entire year. Before this time, I would read every single day. I would be early for work intentionally, just so that I could sit in my car for fifteen minutes with my nose buried in one book or another. It was my way of preparing myself for the day ahead.

Nothing seemed to really hold my interest anymore. I would go home, collapse into bed, and just turn into a zombie. Then, I would sleep until it was time to get up and go to work again. That was the entire scope of my life. Just rinse and repeat.

Even my days off were spent hiding out from the world. Sometimes, I would manage to do a few chores around the house, but that was all I had the energy to accomplish.

You would think, at some point, that I would have realized something was very wrong. However, one thing we nurses excel at is the art of stuffing. No matter what horrible events might occur, there is nothing that can't be repressed if we stomp down on it hard enough. Just take those crappy old feelings and put 'em somewhere deep down, where they will never be heard from again. Why confront our emotions when they can be ignored instead?

Much simpler. What's that old saying? "Physician, heal thyself (and nurses too)." Yeah, we don't really do that.

Ignoring problems sounds like a very healthy way to deal with things, does it not? After all, if we pretend something doesn't exist, it vanishes from existence like a puff of smoke. Of course it does. Apparently, this is not the case. I know, I was as shocked as you are when I found out. In my case, it was becoming increasingly obvious that I was not ok. The warning signs were all there, and a catastrophe was coming at me like a speeding train. Pretending that everything is ok only works until it doesn't anymore.

Of course, no emotional pain is complete without some inappropriate coping mechanisms. I have always been a bit of a joker, but I started to make a joke out of everything. For several weeks, I went through a phase where I would put funny signs up on the doors every few days. One was a "closed" sign that I put up on the doors leading in from the ambulance bay. Another time, I put a "please use other door" sign up on the front door and another one on the back door. They only stayed up for long enough to get a picture (I'm not that dumb, after all). I thought that these pranks were hilarious, but underneath the mirth there was an underlying frustration that was very real. I really did want to put a closed sign up when I was working, just to give the staff a break. No matter what we did, or how busy we got, people just kept coming in. I would have done anything to break that cycle.

Another time, one of our doctors was going to see a patient. He went into the wrong room without realizing what he had done. Instead of enquiring about the patient's name, he bravely forged ahead and performed a full assessment. Eventually, he emerged, thinking his job was complete. That is when I informed him that his actual patient was in the *next* room. He had just wasted twenty minutes of his time. For the rest of the shift, every time he had another patient, I would leave big notes on the doors for him. They would say either "no, not this one" or "this way" with a big arrow on it.

. . .

About a year before I left, the nightmares began. I am not talking about once in a while either. No, I was treated to bad dreams on a nightly basis. They always had the same three themes.

The first theme was the most frequent. I would be in a huge room, just full of sick people, and I would have to look after all of them. In most of the dreams, I would start doing something for one patient that would normally only take a few minutes. Suddenly, I would realize that twelve hours had gone by. My shift was almost over, and I had not even seen any of the other patients. The location would change, but it was always some type of giant warehouse.

Sometimes, the theme would alter just a little. Before becoming a nurse, I had worked mostly in restaurants as a cook. Occasionally, in my dreams, I would find myself attempting to cook for too many people at once. It was the same idea of not being able to keep up, just in a different setting.

There were even a few times that I would dream about my ex-wife. I would be dropping her off at work, and it would be the same warehouse.

The second theme involved me being at work and going on my break. I would go outside or walk through a door, and suddenly I would find myself miles away from the hospital with no way to get back. The rest of the dream would be spent frantically trying to return, but never being able to.

In the third kind of nightmare, I would be working with a doctor on a critical patient. The doctor would be yelling at me to bring him things, but I wouldn't be able to understand what he was saying. I would just stand there, helplessly, not knowing what to do. This dream has become much more frequent of late.

Due to the nightmares, we can add not sleeping to my list of symptoms. I would often wake up several times a night. When I did manage to stay asleep, I was still very restless. As a result, I would still get up feeling exhausted, as though I hadn't really slept at all. Fun times. After all, who really needs to sleep anyway? Certainly not nurses, who can kill people when we aren't paying attention to what we are doing. What could possibly go wrong?

I managed to get through an entire year like this, somehow.

Meanwhile, my fellow nurses were dropping like flies. I think that there is a certain tipping point in any type of job. It comes when too many of the senior staff move on at the same time, which causes the rest of the senior staff to burn out even faster. More people leave, which in turn puts even greater pressure on the ones that remain behind. It eventually becomes a self-perpetuating cycle. Think about it. If you had an extra task that needed doing, are you likely to give it to the new person who is already struggling, or to the seasoned employee? The problem in this scenario is that we assume the experienced employee is not also struggling. They are often just hiding it better, or they are simply more resigned to the whole situation. Whatever the reason, I found myself bearing an even heavier load as the number of new staff members increased around me.

Into this mix, we must also include mentorship. New staff require help and not just with physical tasks. They also require information. They need guidance when faced with situations they are not familiar with. As it turns out, the training that they receive doesn't cover everything. Now, this is not to say that the new people are annoying or a burden in any way. I actually love that part of the job. It does become a time-consuming activity, however. When you are expending so much energy simply trying to keep up with your own work, it becomes just another drain on your already depleted resources. At times, I would find myself resenting the newcomers.

The worst part is that the new people know this. They can often start to feel that they *are* a burden. As a result, they become hesitant to interrupt with questions that they might have. That is how mistakes happen. There were a few times that I would notice one of them doing something the wrong way. Often, when they were already halfway through whatever task they were working on.

For example, there was an elderly patient who came in having a stroke (unlike mine, it was a real one). I was busy with my own patient load, so I just tried to keep an eye on the situation. The doctor quickly came and assessed the patient. He decided that the patient would be given a medication that breaks down clots, allowing circulation to be restored to the affected area of the brain. The primary nurse was fairly new. He began to prepare the medication, and he was joined by a second new staff member who had offered to help. The instructions are printed out, so all they had to do was follow along with each step. Once they were ready to go, one of them asked me if I could check on what they had done. As it turned out, it was very lucky that they did. Even though they had followed the procedure to the letter, they had used the wrong instruction sheet. We have a different protocol for those over a certain age, because they require a reduced dose. Giving the medication as we would to someone younger increases the risk of bleeding, which can be life threatening.

Afterwards, of course, I end up feeling bad when things like this occur. Not because I had made a mistake, but because a mistake was almost made nonetheless. This could have ended very differently, all because I did not have the time to provide proper guidance.

During this period, I did make one decision that I felt really good about. I told the managers that I would no longer do charge nurse shifts. I realized that running the department had become a no-win situation. Being in charge meant having all the responsibility without having any of the authority. As the situation in our department continued to deteriorate, that sense of powerlessness only increased. No one seemed to have any solutions. No one seemed to be planning ahead. The charge nurses were just expected to deal with it.

There seemed to be a systemic acceptance of our situation, like everyone was just resigned to this fate. When our numbers first began to climb, management would often involve themselves directly. We would see them scurrying everywhere, trying to remedy the overcrowding. They would go from floor to floor, bed to bed, facilitating discharges for people who were able to go home. After a while, though, that effort just petered out. Soon, the only response we would get seemed to be a shrug of the shoulders and an "oh, well." Once management has given up, the staff will not be far behind because we look to them for guidance. They set the tone. Without hope, morale tends to crumble very quickly.

The worst part is once someone gets into that mindset, all they can focus on is reacting. Twice a day, all the charge nurses would get together with management and attempt to plan out the day. I can remember attending such a meeting once, discussing where we were going to put everyone. At these meetings, it often appeared like we were discussing some sort of giant Rubik's Cube. Somehow, if we just shuffled the patients around enough, empty beds would miraculously appear. Anyway, at this particular meeting, we had somehow managed to find a space for every patient that needed one. We had avoided a disaster for another day. At the end of the meeting, I piped up. "Well, this is great. What's our plan for next week?" Everyone just looked at me. A few gave me the shrug. The meeting was over.

This is exactly what I meant earlier when I talked about preventing a crisis before it happens. To accomplish that, there needs to be a group of people committed to *anticipating* problems, instead of simply reacting to them. They can then proactively enact solutions so that we never reach a crisis point. By doing this, we wouldn't have to constantly be playing catch-up. This doesn't seem to occur to anyone in authority where I work. If it did, the last three years of my life might have gone very differently.

THE BIG DAY

Now, we have arrived at "the day." You might be wondering why I put the quotation marks in there. Well, like any good storyteller, I am going to tell you. Whenever we talk about emotional trauma and post-traumatic stress, everyone becomes obsessed with talking about "the day." It's as if all the days before and after suddenly cease to exist, and that one singular moment becomes the reason for everything that happens. As someone who has lived through the experience, I am here to tell you that this is just not the case.

The simple truth is that I had been sitting on a cliff edge for over a year. The events of "the day" simply gave me a nudge, and over the precipice I went. This is not to downplay what happened that day or to minimize it in any way. I am simply saying that the events of that day did not happen in isolation. They were the culmination of a lot of days. It's like going on a trip. No one suddenly appears at their destination. First, there is a journey that we must take.

On this particular day, I was orienting a new employee to the department. It was our last set of shifts together, so she was doing most of the work herself. As a result, I was considered "extra" (there's those quotation marks again). Our charge nurse that day has a reputation for being a real shit magnet. Whenever she was on, you could always expect something really bad to happen, like a bus full of seniors overturning. Often, it would be more than one something. She certainly didn't disappoint us on this shift.

The first case I worked on was a woman who had come from one of the care homes. She came to our section, but my orientee was busy, so I stepped in to help. The woman had been sent in for something very minor. It turned out that she was, in fact, critical. To make matters worse, no one had sent along her code status, so we had to give her the full meal deal, right from the beginning (without knowing someone's wishes, we have to assume that they want us to do everything). Luckily, a family member arrived about an hour into it and told us that we could stop what we were doing. She did have a do-not-resuscitate order in place. We did stop everything, and she died about three hours later. It began as an intense experience, but it ended rather peacefully. I would have managed just fine if that had been the only such occurrence. Unfortunately, the day was just getting started.

Just after the first patient had passed away, one of the other nurses received a small child that we see quite frequently. He has a genetic disorder, and he is often very sick when he comes in. Even when he looks well, his condition can still deteriorate rapidly. This day was no exception, of course. The nurse that was looking after him was also fairly new, so I was again called in to assist. If it takes a new nurse a long time to feel comfortable, it takes even more time to be comfortable looking after children. The patient was not doing well at all. Because of his disorder, his care was both extensive and complicated, and we decided he could be better managed in the trauma room. Here, we had better access to any equipment we might need. We would also be able to provide him with one-to-one care. I was the only nurse available to go with him, so off I went.

It took some time, and a great deal of work, but I did manage to get him settled eventually. He wasn't out of the woods, but he appeared to be improving at least. Now, we were just waiting for one of the pediatricians to come down and admit him. Even though things had calmed down by this point, I was still feeling some stress. Working with little ones always takes an emotional toll, so my nerves were already frazzled. I was relieved because he was out of immediate danger. I also felt very sad, however, because I knew that this little guy had already spent a great deal of his life in the hospital. The mom had as well.

I must explain something at this point. Otherwise, the rest of the story will not make sense. We were supposed to have two triage nurses that day. However, one of our triage nurses had a student with him. This nurse has always been a bit of a trauma junkie, so he is always trying to get in on whatever is most exciting. Having a student with him only made this propensity worse, as he wanted the student to see everything. To be fair, triage is a very boring place for students. There's nothing for them to do but watch. Still, there is nothing worse than working at triage with a partner who continually wanders off, which is exactly what this nurse had been doing. Because of this, our other triage nurse (I shall call her Duine Gearr) had been working more or less alone for the entire day. She would ask him to come back to the triage area, which he would do for a little while. He would remain there for the shortest possible time he thought he could get away with. Then, he would toddle off again. She was getting angrier and angrier as the day wore on. I could see the frustration on her face.

Now, where was I? Yes, I was in the trauma room looking after child number one. There was an elderly gentleman in the second trauma bay. Suddenly, Duine Gearr ran in. She informed me that another sick child had just arrived. She was going to stay and get the trauma room prepared, and she asked me to go out to the triage desk so that I could bring this new patient in.

Now, we both faced difficult choices, impossible choices really. She was alone at triage. We had no idea where the second triage nurse was. Therefore, she was forced to decide whether to abandon the triage desk and a waiting room full of people in order to look after this child. She also had to make a space in the trauma room, which necessitated moving the elderly gentleman out into the hallway, with no one to look after him. He needed to be on a monitor, but no others were available, so she just had to leave him there.

I was faced with the choice of having to desert one sick child in order to deal with another, sicker child. Those are the kinds of choices we are forced to make on a daily basis, because we are never provided with the resources we require in order to do things properly.

Anyway, I went out to the triage desk. Luckily, by this point the other triage nurse had returned to his post.

When I first saw our new patient, I swear to God, I thought the kid had died right there. He was the most awful shade of gray-blue, and his respirations were very shallow. Mom held the little boy in her arms, and the child just lay there, limply. I should explain that children are very different from adults when they are sick or hurt. Adults decline steadily, children decline like they are dropping off a cliff. There is no sight more terrifying to an ER nurse than a floppy child, because it means that the child is physically exhausted and is rapidly running out of resources. They are nearing the point when the body will just give up. I grabbed mom and literally pushed her into the trauma room.

Once in the trauma room, we got the patient on the stretcher and started hooking him up to the monitor. At this point, Duine Gearr started to cry. She was completely overwhelmed, not by the patient, but by the frustration and anger she had been feeling all day. It all caught up to her in that moment.

I won't go into details, except to say that this child was very, very ill. To make matters worse, there were things that had to be done right away to save his life, and we didn't have the time to be nice about it. This, of course, made him even more distressed and frightened. He was too young to really understand what we were doing and why. All he knew was that a group of total strangers was trying to hurt him. I had to hold down his head as the doctor performed a very painful procedure, one that needed to be performed immediately. I do not even know how to describe the many emotions that I was feeling in that moment. There is fear, certainly. That is obvious. More subtle, or perhaps just harder to explain, is the overwhelming sense of guilt that came over me. It always does whenever I am faced with a scenario such as this. Consciously, I know that there is an immediate need to save the child's life, and this overrides every other consideration. Somewhere deep down, however, is the knowledge that I am forcibly pinning a child's head to the stretcher while we do horrible things to him. He is screaming in terror while we intentionally cause him a great deal of pain. There is no logic to this feeling, but it is still there nonetheless. Hurting a child goes against every instinct that I possess as a nurse and as a human being. It takes an enormous amount of effort not to start screaming.

It was obvious that the patient needed to be flown out to another hospital immediately. Again, we are simply not equipped to deal with some types of patients, and children in critical condition are certainly within that category. He needed the experts. While we waited for the helicopter to come and take him, the team continued their work. At this point, I stepped out. We had performed the most critical tasks already, so they no longer needed me there. I was told later that, after I had left the room, he had gotten even worse. It seems that the steps we had taken to save his life earlier had also made his condition more acute. This is not to say that we had made mistakes. Each of those steps had been absolutely necessary to take at the time. Again, it's about difficult choices, and sometimes we have to do things that are bad in order to prevent things that are worse. If we hadn't done exactly what we did, he would most likely have died right there. We had given him a chance at least. However, once again that irrational feeling of guilt rears up, as if it is somehow our fault that his condition is getting worse.

One of the worst parts of working in this particular ER was that we almost never find out what happens to our patients. We would just do our bit, and then they would go elsewhere. There are certain patients that really rip out your insides, but we are consistently left without any real sense of closure. To this day, I have no idea if that little boy survived. That sense of not knowing the outcome can make the emotional impact so much worse.

Of course, this horrendous day was not over yet. No, the universe had one last surprise for me. As I came out of the trauma room, there was a woman yelling out for help in the lobby. Apparently, she needed help getting her husband out of the car.

Now, remember a while back when I told the story of my first code blue? Well, this was déjà vu. Hubby was slumped over in the passenger seat, barely breathing. He was also very pale. We somehow managed to get him out of the car and onto a stretcher. Then we pushed him inside and directly into a room. Woosh, woosh. He was on the monitor, he had an IV, and we were ready to go. We worked desperately to save him, but it was obvious that he was going downhill fast. His body was giving up. Moreover, he was quite elderly, so our chances of bringing him back at that point were as close to zero as they get. The doctor had a quick word with the wife, and he laid out the options for her. He also told her what her husband's chances were. She gave us permission to stop and he passed away only a few minutes later. I am just glad that, this time, we hadn't dragged it out unnecessarily. It must be so difficult to make such a decision in the heat of the moment like that, but I was thankful to her for making it. Sometimes there is nothing we can do to halt the dying process and trying to can often feel worse, both for us and for the family.

After someone dies, there is a great deal of paperwork that has to be filled out. What would a hospital be without a whole lot of paperwork? We also have to prepare the patient for the morgue (I will spare you the details). In the case of the first patient, my orientee was the nurse. In the last case, the nurse was also brand new to the ER. Because of this, it was left to me to complete all the paperwork in both cases. Neither of them knew how. I did show them all the steps to take, but I had to do most of the work myself. In the second case, this necessitated staying about half an hour past shift change, as if the day had not been long enough already.

After all of this, I was talking with Duine Gearr behind the triage desk. We were comparing notes, and it turned out that we were having many of the same symptoms. Anger, poor sleep, etc. After a year and a half, I had become a real expert at ignoring what was going on with me, so I had never stopped to connect the dots before. Then, she said something that blew me out of the water. "That sounds just like PTSD" I was shocked. The thought that what I had been experiencing was more than just stress had simply never even occurred to me. Just the idea that my emotional state had a name was a total revelation. In that moment, everything that I had been experiencing for the last year began to make some measure of sense.

I went home that day and just collapsed on my bed. I felt like a truck had rolled over my body. There was just this deep, empty pit inside of me. I felt so totally done. As it turns out, just like my last patient of the day, my body was giving up too. It knew when to quit before I did.

...

The next day I got up as usual. I got ready, grabbed my lunch, and headed out the door. It seemed just like any other day. The drive was uneventful, and as I pulled into the parking lot, I was feeling fine. There was nothing out of the ordinary, nothing to warn me of what was coming.

I got out of the car and headed for the main door into the emergency room. That's when someone decided to drop a load of bricks right on top of my chest. I couldn't breathe, my heart was racing, I was drenched in sweat, and my hands were shaking. Thankfully, I had seen symptoms like these enough to know what was happening or I might have thought I was having a heart attack (much like my stroke earlier). I had just experienced my first panic attack. I stood outside for several minutes, willing myself to calm down.

I did manage to go inside eventually, once I had gotten my emotions in check. Looking back, I probably should have called it quits, right then and there. For a few years before this, I had always experienced a sense of dread when I came to work. Sometimes it had been very hard going inside when I already knew that it was going to be another awful day. This was entirely different. I had never felt genuine fear before. In fact, being an ER nurse, I did not even think that the word fear was in my vocabulary. What made me continue inside was thinking that I would be able to take it easy for the day. I could let my orientee do most of the work. No such luck. The department was chock-full of people, all the beds were full, and we were working in the ambulatory area. There were more than enough patients to keep us both busy.

There is a phenomenon in our department that we call creeping. It happens whenever our stretchers are all full. This causes the acuity level in streaming to go up, simply because there is nowhere else for patients to go. The very definition of ambulatory is to be able to walk. When creeping begins, however, that can become a very loose definition. Anyone who can stand at all, no matter how wobbly they might be when doing so, gets sent over to the ambulatory area. In other words, ambulatory starts to fill up with some very inappropriate patients on days like this.

To make matters worse, I was working with Duine Gearr again. This meant that both of our stress levels were already quite high, right from the start of the day. Neither of us was in the mood to take anyone's crap.

The morning passed by very quickly, due to the sheer volume of patients we had. It was during the afternoon, however, that things really started to fall apart. My orientee, Duine Gearr, and I were struggling with some very sick patients, all at the same time.

I had a patient who was going through alcohol withdrawal. He was in really rough shape: shaking, sweating, pasty. It was instantly obvious that he was very close to full-blown DTs, which is a condition that long-time alcoholics get when they suddenly stop drinking. There is a 10 percent mortality rate, so it can be quite serious. In the back of my mind, I was already well aware that this was going to go badly. Fortunately, that meant that I was prepared for what happened next. As soon as I poked him with the IV needle, he started having a seizure. We quickly moved him in to one of the exam rooms, where I managed to keep him safe until the seizure subsided. I also gave him some medication to prevent further seizures. After ensuring that he was improving, we had him moved to a monitored spot. That is most definitely where he should have gone to begin with.

At the same time that my patient was crashing, Duine Gearr was having to contend with a patient with a rapid heart rate. He had a pulse of 130, and there was no chance that we would be able to deal with that appropriately in the ambulatory area. There is not one heart monitor over there. He needed a monitored bed right away, just as my guy had only moments before. Duine Gearr was absolutely livid because of what was going on.

Immediately after we got the second patient moved over, we had need of a third bed. My orientee's patient was crashing in one of the exam rooms. She was having some respiratory distress and was getting much worse. Medication was not working. She ended up being intubated and sent to the ICU only a short time later. If a patient from ambulatory ends up going to the ICU, it is a safe bet that they should not have been sent to ambulatory in the first place. Remember, again, we have no way of monitoring such patients over there.

At this point, I was turning into a total basket case. All I could manage to feel in those moments was frustration and anger. I had to leave the floor to go and cry. That's when I had my second panic attack. Apparently, I was on a roll that day.

This is when the realization truly hit me. I knew that I was done. I went and talked to the department manager and told her exactly what was happening. I was very close to crying right there in her office. I then informed her that I would try and finish out the set, as my orientee only had two more shifts after that. However, after I had completed those two shifts, I would not be returning. She understood and was very supportive of my decision. Maybe she simply realized that neither of us had a choice in the matter any longer. I was either going to leave voluntarily, or I was going to collapse.

Now, in theory, I had the next two shifts all planned out. They were both night shifts, so they should not have been as busy. I arranged for my orientee and I to be in the monitored area, because I knew that she could carry the whole load on her own over there. My job, again in theory, was just to watch and help out. Unfortunately, I was an emotional mess for both shifts, and I'm not entirely sure that I was any help at all.

I was making mistakes on things that I had done a thousand times in the past. My ability to concentrate on anything had completely evaporated. It felt as though I was forgetting every single thing. As an example, I was starting an IV on a patient and I forgot to clamp it. That was something I had never forgotten before. Without the clamp on, the IV tubing is open to the outside. Blood ended up going everywhere. There were a few other episodes that were similar to this one.

At about 3 a.m. on the second night shift, I felt another panic attack coming on. There was an elderly woman in the hallway who kept moaning loudly, over and over. Just the thought of a patient having to suffer like that in the hall, where all the world could see her, was really grating on my nerves (not the patient, the situation). To make it worse, the buzzers were all buzzing, and the monitors were all beeping. All that noise just overwhelmed me. Suddenly, I felt as if the entire world was closing in, crushing me down. All I could think of in that moment was escape.

I talked to the charge nurse and told her that I had to leave right away because I knew that I could not stand a moment more. That was my last official shift.

HOW TO LOSE YOUR MIND
IN THREE EASY STEPS

If someone breaks a leg at work, the whole process for reporting and receiving compensation for said injury is rather simple. After all, breaking your leg is not unusual. The whole system is designed for people who break a leg. As a result, the steps are laid out for the injured party and are easy to follow.

When you break your brain at work, things become a little more complicated.

The day after I had left work, my first call was to NATH. Then I called my employer's injury reporting line. After that, I had no idea what I was supposed to do next. Who was I supposed to call?

One thing that I think most people do not fully appreciate is just how exhausting mental health conditions can be. Some days are good, and I can get all my tasks accomplished. Often, however, my big accomplishment for the day is getting the dishes done. Sometimes, even getting out of bed seems like too much of a chore. I never know what the day will be like until I actually get moving. I never know what my energy level is going to be. It certainly takes a lot of getting used to, especially as I am accustomed to being a high functioning individual. At first, it was as if the universe had given me an entirely new personality. I had to learn how to let things go and to celebrate the little achievements, rather than obsessing over what I hadn't managed to do. If I can only get one thing done during the day, I have now reached a point where I can be ok with that. It's all about being kind to myself. I must now accept my new limitations.

You can imagine what it was like when I first went off work, though. I had all these things that I had to figure out on my own, but no energy to do any of them. Also, my entire thinking process was dysfunctional at that point. Everything seemed to be so much harder to deal with. Trying to figure out a difficult process under these circumstances can get somewhat surreal because my own brain seemed unwilling to cooperate with the process. Yet, there was really no one to help with any of this. I remember getting calls from people six months later, asking why I had not informed them of what had happened. My union, for example. How was I supposed to know, though? With the state I was in, I was just doing the best I could to muddle through.

I did attempt to contact various psychologists right away. I did not enjoy riding on the emotional roller coaster, so I was very motivated to get an appointment as soon as possible. The earliest appointment I could find was ten months away. Take a moment to think about that, if you will. Ten months? For someone having an acute mental health crisis, the earliest appointment was in ten months. I wasn't sleeping, I was super anxious all the time, and I would jump ten feet into the air every time a siren went by. My entire world was coming apart at the seams, and I really had no one with whom to talk about it on a professional level. I wanted solutions.

There are crisis centers around here, and I did access some of those. However, crisis centers are designed specifically for people in crisis. In other words, they were great to talk to if I was having a panic attack, but they had no real answers for me in regard to my actual condition.

After the event with the sick child, the hospital did provide a counsellor who was proficient in critical incident debriefing. It felt immensely unhelpful, however. My work has a contract with an outside agency, and whenever we had a critical incident, they would send someone to talk to us. The people that they send, however, have no medical background at all. They certainly have no idea what it is like to work in an ER. Their entire approach tends to be a rather generic one. It was as if someone had given the debriefer a script to read at some point, and she was just repeating it. We were told to get more rest, drink more water, and go for walks. Meanwhile, I'm sitting there having a deep emotional crisis, while the rest of the staff are literally on the verge of tears. It was much like having an arm chopped off and having someone show up to help with a Band-Aid and some Polysporin. Afterwards, I was talking with the debriefer. She actually congratulated me on recognizing the symptoms of PTSD in myself. You will recall that I had *not* recognized the signs at all, or not until it was far too late at least. I informed her that she was mistaken about me. She again told me to drink more water.

After a few weeks, I did manage to get in to see a therapist, at least. I had seen her previously through my work. She had helped me during my marriage difficulties, so I was already comfortable with her. However, there were problems with this process as well. The rules prohibited her from doing any treatments for the Post-traumatic stress disorder, because she was not registered with NATH. This, despite the fact that she was a registered trauma counselor. It was still enormously helpful just to have someone to talk to. Holding all these emotions in for so long was making life very unpleasant for me. I felt like I was going to explode at any moment. Still, it would have been a lot more productive for my state of mind if we could have started effective treatments right away. In any case, I was only allowed a few sessions with her. I had already used up my allotted visits through work, so I had to apply for some free visits through another agency. I was approved, but they could only give me a few sessions.

I should probably describe what was going on for me, emotionally, at this time. Post-traumatic stress disorder (PTSD) is a condition that happens as the result of an emotional trauma. Normally, when an ordinary event happens to us, our subconscious takes it in and processes it. The event then gets moved to our long-term memory while we sleep. Sometimes, however, an event happens that is beyond the ability of the subconscious to process. When this occurs, that event essentially becomes stuck in short-term memory. It's sort of like a skipping record (for those of you that can remember what a record is). The person becomes stuck in that moment, replaying it over and over again. Therefore, that fear we feel in moments of high stress becomes stuck as well. The person with PTSD is literally unable to get past it.

Essentially, I was in fight or flight mode, twenty-four seven. That feeling never subsided. I woke up anxious, I went to bed anxious, and I was anxious all day in between. It felt like I was constantly waiting for something bad to happen. If you can remember a time that someone snuck up behind you to scare you, that's what I felt like all day, every day. They call this state hypervigilance.

Just to make it even more fun, there were still the nightmares to contend with. They continued to haunt me virtually every night. I was getting hardly any sleep at all. Then there were the dissociative episodes, which I have already described. Thankfully, they do not happen often. I also found it very difficult to concentrate on simple tasks. For instance, even watching TV was a challenge because I couldn't follow the plot most of the time. Trying to read anything longer than a birthday card was impossible.

One common symptom that I did not experience personally was guilt. Sometimes, there is a feeling that the person with PTSD could have done something differently. "If only I had…" You would see this, for instance, with sexual assault victims. Often, they can feel as if the rape was somehow their fault. For me, it was more a feeling of powerlessness, that I had no control over the events that had occurred. Instead of feeling shame, I felt a great deal of anger toward a system that I believed had failed me. I had simply done the best that I could in an impossible situation. It is a good thing that I am a confident person, at least when it comes to my nursing skills. Otherwise, I think it would have been very easy to spiral downward into despair, to think that I had done this to myself. As it was, I knew exactly whom to hold responsible.

In the beginning, I did experience a great deal of depression. I will be honest here and tell you that I did experience suicidal thoughts frequently, for the first few months. In fact, to be even more open, I still do have such thoughts. Very rarely now, though. The funny thing is, it wasn't because of the depression, or maybe it wasn't *just* because of the depression. It was more just wanting the constant anxiety to end. I came to resent the fact that every day was now exactly the same. Nothing improved. I not only felt crappy all the time, but I also could see no end to it at all. Every day was filled with nothing but anxiety. Knowing that tomorrow will not bring any relief takes away hope, and that lack of hope sucks the life right out of a person. I would break down in tears at least once a day.

The irony is that what really kept me going from day to day was being a health care worker. I knew that if I did kill myself, it would have been someone I know who would have found me afterwards. The paramedics who would have had to come to my house and the nurses and doctors who would have had to try and save me, these are all friends of mine. The last thing I wanted to do was inflict that kind of emotional trauma on them. There were likely a few who might not have been too upset to see me go, but I'm hoping that it wasn't the majority (squints at friends). I especially didn't want to be the cause of someone else's PTSD. Besides, who wants to be seen by friends after they've pooped yourself or worse.

I did manage to get in to see my own doctor right away, which was nice. She is so great. She is one of those physicians who actually listens to her patients. I cannot even begin to describe how grateful I am to have her as my doctor. I would not have made it through those first few months without her. The funny thing is that I had kind of stumbled into being her patient by accident. In my area, family doctors are at a premium. I had searched high and low for years. Finally, I found one who had just moved to the area. Unfortunately, he really wasn't very good. For example, I have chronic knee pain, especially in the winter. The meniscus in my right knee has a tear. He once told me that the solution was to walk more. Now, being a nurse in the ER, I probably walk the equivalent of a hike across Russia every single shift. Perhaps you can begin to appreciate why I didn't find that little tidbit helpful in the least. Luckily, he retired fairly soon after he arrived here. My current doctor then took over his patients.

During that first visit after my meltdown, she made sure that I was able to remain off from work. She also put me on medication right away. A combination of antidepressants and a medication for nightmares. Though the meds didn't make the feelings go away entirely, they certainly helped. The endless sadness seemed to ease up, at least. I didn't feel like crying all the time anymore.

The drug to reduce my nightmares was an absolute godsend. Seriously, it was life changing. If you have nightmares related to post-traumatic stress, you need this stuff. I went from having bad dreams every night to maybe having them once a week. My sleep patterns still suck, but at least I'm not waking up twenty times a night in terror anymore. Now, if only I could actually fall asleep to begin with, everything would be great.

The one drawback of this drug is that it was originally designed as a blood pressure medication. My blood pressure tends toward the low side to begin with. I have to be really careful about getting up too fast if I have to pee in the middle of the night. I'm sure all the older guys reading this will sympathize with me here. If I have to get up in the middle of the night to pee, I'm really not thinking about doing it slowly at that point. It is usually somewhat urgent.

I recently had a bout of bronchitis, and I had to stop taking the nightmare medication for a week. Every time I coughed, everything would go rather dark for a minute or two. I came very close to passing out a few times.

Still, I was so grateful to my doctor for prescribing this medication. I have no idea how she even knew about it, as the medication is not meant to be used in this way. Instead, it is a little-known side effect, or what we call an off-label use. That's how good she is.

In sharp contrast to my doctor, there were others who were not helpful in the least. NATH was downright brutal to me after I had opened my claim. It took a couple of weeks before anyone even contacted me.

Once they had, the first thing that my caseworker did was conduct a phone interview. This involved having me live through the entire day of my trauma, all over again. Even now, working on that last chapter was very difficult for me. I actually ended up bawling my eyes out in the middle of a crowded restaurant while I was writing it. It has been over a year and a half since that day, yet the wound is obviously still raw. Now, just imagine what it was like after only a few weeks, when the events were still fresh in my mind. Add to this the fact that I could sense her lack of empathy in the tone of her voice.

After I was finished talking, she proceeded to ask me the most insensitive questions I have ever been asked. When we were talking about the young boy, she actually had the temerity to ask me, "Well, did he die?" First off, that is entirely irrelevant. Any time we have a patient who is actively trying to die on us, it is traumatic. It really makes no difference if the patient actually dies or not. This is even more true when the patient is a small child. Second, you have to remember that this woman was simply my caseworker. She was in no way qualified to make any psychological assessment of me or of my condition. Her job should be to find me a trained professional. Someone proficient in psychology should be deciding the validity of me claim, not her. Trying to quantify my emotional trauma to this woman was not only extremely hard on me, it was actually harmful. I spent most of the rest of the day curled up in a ball on the floor, shaking.

There's also the added stress of having to watch what I say and how much I divulge. As a nurse, I still have to consider confidentiality. As a result, I had to walk a very fine line between providing enough information to satisfy her questions, while also trying not to say too much. That's hard to accomplish, considering how upsetting the entire conversation was.

Essentially, the caseworker's attitude was that, yes, that day had sucked. However, my workplace always sucked, so there was nothing different about that particular day. I spent months having her tell me that it was doubtful my claim would be approved, for that very reason. The diagnosis of PTSD, according to NATH, had to involve an event that was totally outside the normal parameters of my work. Since I worked in an ER, crappy was just to be expected. Even trying to save a critically ill child was considered "normal," apparently. In other words, I couldn't possibly have been stressed because I work in a place where there is always a great deal of stress.

But that's not really what PTSD is all about. In fact, NATH's definition differs significantly from the definition of PTSD used by the entire rest of the world! Yes, it usually does revolve around one particular event. However, this completely discounts the fact that there is also a cumulative effect, and that this can play a very important role in PTSD. Their definition also fails to take into account that, while most of our days are crappy in the ER, some days are crappy times ten. I'm sure their definition is right though, because they're the experts. After all, what do all those mental health professionals know anyway? Their definition of PTSD seemed to exist for the sole purpose of rejecting anyone making a claim for PTSD. It was like breaking a leg at work and then having someone with no medical training try to tell me that it's not really broken.

Me: "Look, there's little bits of bone sticking out."

Them: "No there isn't. You're just imagining it."

Me: "But it's bending the wrong way."

Them: "Quit faking."

Keep in mind that I was not receiving any pay during most of this period. I did receive some sick pay in the beginning, but that ran out quickly. After that, my work gave me two weeks' pay in lieu of my NATH claim. In other words, I would have to pay them back as soon as I received benefits. The same benefits that I was still not sure I was going to receive. There's nothing like seeing a negative balance on a paycheck, particularly when I was not sure I would have any money coming in. I could easily have ended up owing my work a few thousand dollars out of my own pocket.

Just to add to the absurdity of the whole situation, I was still unable to access any sort of professional counselling while I was waiting for my claim to be approved. I ended up in a holding pattern for months. With NATH, nothing ever happens quickly. They move with all the speed of a very large rock. That is, of course, until they need *me* to do something. Then it's all "hurry up" and "why wasn't this done yesterday?"

Have I mentioned that they kept losing one of my forms, as well? That was super special fun. It wasn't just any old form either. It was a letter of consent, so that they could access all my medical records. They needed this in order to move forward with my claim, so it was kind of vital to the process. I sent it six times in total. I faxed it, I mailed it, I sent it by registered mail. Apparently, it kept ending up in the same place that socks go in the dryer. I even faxed it directly to the office of my caseworker, and they still managed to misplace it! If it had not been happening to me, this whole thing would have been quite funny. Because it *was* happening to me, it really wasn't funny at all. In the end, I had to take it directly to the branch office here in town. I then had to stand at the desk and watch them as they scanned it into my file. I wasn't about to trust any of them at that point.

. . .

The hardest part of this entire experience was sitting still. I don't do time off very well. You will recall that when I hurt my back, I pretty much had to be forced from the department. After a few weeks of being at home with nothing to do, I was getting very restless. Now, I had nothing to fill my time, and it was driving me absolutely bonkers. Worse, I was alone with my thoughts all the time. Depression and boredom do not mix very well. A bored mind starts to look for things to obsess over, which only makes the depression worse. I also couldn't relieve the boredom by going outside, due to the anxiety I was feeling.

Also, I don't think anyone was able to fully understand just how much of a lifestyle change this entailed. I used to be an emergency nurse. I am used to being someone who is high functioning, always in control. I was the person who was cool in a crisis. I walked with confidence everywhere I went. Often, I would get stopped in stores by other shoppers who wanted to ask me questions. Once, when I inquired why someone had assumed I was an employee, she replied that I just looked like I belonged there. That was my life before this.

My therapist once pointed out that there are many people who feel stress at levels that are inappropriate. He went on to add that, just as I now experience stress at a higher level, there are those who always feel stress at a lower level than others. In other words, risk-takers. He said it like it was a foreign concept to me, until I pointed out that I had fit into *that* category before all of this had happened. I think that was the first time that he really understood what I was talking about when I described how much my life had changed. It wasn't just that my anxiety level had risen, it was that I had really gone from one extreme to the other. These days, I would be quite happy if I could just settle in the middle somewhere.

Now, I am anxious literally all the time. I have absolutely no control over my emotions anymore. Loud noises have me running for cover. Last Christmas, my girlfriend at the time was baking cookies. Just having the stove beeping when the cookies were done was triggering me. I even had to change the ringtone on my phone to something more soothing. Any time I received a phone call, it just about scared me to death.

Essentially, I had lost me. My entire self-identity was in tatters, and no one seemed in a rush to help me find it again. Every aspect of my life was irreparably altered to the point that I didn't even recognize my life anymore. Because of this, I experienced a profound sense of grief and loss. It was almost like losing a loved one, only it was my former self that had died. I imagine that soldiers who lose a limb must go through a very similar experience. In the end, it might seem like such a small thing. To me, it was everything. It was who I was.

I realize that I should not feel this way. After all, I am not just my job, so I am told. In reality, I am the job, because the job is me. I chose this career specifically because it was me. Now it is gone, and I have no idea how to fill that void. I need to accept that I may never be able to return.

There were even some of my favorite TV shows that I just couldn't watch anymore. That's not an easy thing to give up when I was sitting around at home all day. To be clear, I didn't have to give up on TV entirely. Thank God for that! I did have to be very careful of what I watched, however. Any medical shows (and I am talking the fictional ones here) were right out, obviously. I would end up having panic attacks for the rest of the day. Medical documentary shows were even worse. Sometimes, I even had a hard time with vet shows. Even now, I will often have a pretty strong reaction to these programs, depending on the topic. Seeing a medical show can still have me bawling my eyes out. Things have improved a little bit, though. Some of the cheesier shows I can now watch without as much of a problem.

In the beginning, even shows that included someone just *going* to the hospital were too much for me. I remember once watching a cop show. There was a character that had been brought to the hospital, and it reminded me of a patient I had once treated. That was all it took. I started having intense flashbacks for hours. Afterwards, I can recall thinking that if I was going to have to relive every single horrible event that I had seen in fourteen years, this was definitely going to take a while.

Any show where a child is hurt also has a strong effect on me. For instance, the science fiction show *Falling Skies*. I enjoyed that show so much, I went out and bought the entire series on Blu-Ray. Now, I can't watch it anymore. In the show, the alien invaders kidnap some of the children. The kids then reappear later wearing these big metal things on their backs that are supposed to hook directly into their spines. Sounds really hokey, I know. I have no idea why, but it still had my brain doing laps.

...

The nonsense with NATH continued for over three months. If I had not received my tax return during that time, I would definitely have starved to death. Then again, perhaps that was the point. Great way to cut costs if all your claimants die before you have to give them any money. The ones that don't die probably just give up and go away out of sheer frustration.

The most frustrating thing is that there is an acute nursing shortage going on right now. Yet, here I sit. I am a highly trained and educated specialty nurse. Still, all I could do was wait around for three months. Don't forget, that's just how long it took to get a decision on my claim. By this point, we hadn't even *started* to address my problems yet. To this day, I firmly believe that if I had been able to access some form of treatment in a timely manner, it would have reduced my recovery time significantly. Instead, I have become more and more isolated over time. The symptoms have become far more entrenched. It has gotten to the point that even being outside can make me anxious now. This doesn't even take into account the stress that going through three months of uncertainty put on me.

One of my favorite NATH moments came when I received a letter from my caseworker explaining why my prescription for anxiety medication would not be covered. They gave two reasons. First, they stated that the medication is not used in the treatment of PTSD. It is used to treat anxiety and sleep disturbances. Now, technically they are right. However, I guess that no one really bothered to check, because those all sound like the symptoms of PTSD to me. The second reason they gave was that it can be addictive, and they were concerned because I have a history of drug abuse. This history was thirty years ago, by the way. I was so addicted to this medication that it took me four months to go through thirty of them.

Now, to be totally honest, I should probably point out that NATH was just as new to this entire process as I was. They had only just started to recognize psychiatric injuries in the workplace, so they had not yet formulated a process to deal with these types of claims. They were feeling their way in the dark, just like I was.

For starters, how do they verify the injury? It's fairly easy to tell if someone has a physical injury. There are all sorts of tests for that, X-rays and that sort of thing. A psychiatric injury is a great deal more subjective, however. I can feel a certain way, but those emotions exist for me alone. I can only share them with someone else up to a point; there is nothing visible to see and the other person can't ever feel what I feel.

Also, when I first began the claim process, I am certain that they only had one case manager in that section. She was probably handling all the mental health claims that they had received. If I am right about that, it's no wonder it took so long. Her workload must have been enormous.

Still, having people wait that long for an answer seems counterproductive, to say the least. The longer the wait, the harder it is to get the person (me) back to a functional level. The sense of isolation starts to become ingrained in the subconscious, and if enough time passes, it starts to become comforting. I used to feel lonely a lot when this began. Now, being alone at home makes me feel like a turtle in a shell. I feel safe here. I have never been afraid of change before (I've had a lot of it in my life). Now, walking into new situations scares the hell out of me.

Had I broken my leg, there is no way that NATH would have had me waiting for three months. Can you imagine? I would have been in for treatment right away. I would have seen a physician that very same day. Certainly, no one would have told the doctor that I could not have my leg casted until a caseworker had approved my claim. Had NATH dealt with a broken leg the same way they dealt with my claim, I would never have walked properly again.

After a while, the wait itself also becomes a point of stress, which further impedes progress. How could I even begin to confront the demons that haunted me when I was worried about money all the time. Those three months were not neutral; they actually brought on further harm. In the long run, it has probably taken me much longer to heal because of the wait. That makes my claim more expensive for them, and that makes no sense at all. The craziest part is, I was informed that some claims for PTSD take even longer than mine did.

Finally, after the three months of waiting, NATH did a complete reversal on me. Suddenly, I was assigned a new caseworker, and she was much more understanding. This was the first time I had experienced any hint of empathy at all from NATH. She called me up and promised to put a rush on my claim. She expressed concern, recognizing how tough this process must have been for me. Most importantly, she appeared to believe me. It is amazing what one single moment of acknowledgment can do for a person. That was a huge turnaround. Only a few weeks before, I had essentially been treated as if there was nothing wrong with me at all, when it was obvious to me that *everything* had changed. Suddenly, I had hope again, and things were finally starting to move forward.

The first item on the agenda was to get me in to see a psychologist. The great irony of this was that I was so broke by this point, I very nearly had to cancel the appointment because I had no gas in my car. Being put into a situation such as that by the people who were supposed to be helping me get better is completely absurd. Honestly, if I didn't laugh about it, I would be screaming. I think it was the day before my appointment that I finally received a check from NATH. Talk about coming through at the very last second. Anyway, I did manage to buy some gas so that I could go.

This wasn't a counselling session either. I would have to wait even longer for that. Instead, this was just so someone could officially diagnose me. It was only step one. Once I had seen the psychologist and he had agreed that this was PTSD, only then would I be funded to get actual therapy.

When I first arrived at his office, I was given several questionnaires. I had to fill in about three thousand answers about myself, my mood, and my symptoms. These were in the form of multiple-choice questions, such as "In the last two weeks, have you had any feelings of sadness?" Then I would have to fill in the appropriate circle: one being definitely yes, five being definitely no, and the rest being somewhere in between. Needless to say, after filling in hundreds of little circles for an hour, I was more than a little bored. Plus, now my hand really hurt. At least they hadn't made me bring my own pencil.

After I had completed the forms, I was able to speak with the actual psychologist for a while. He was very kind and soft spoken, and he essentially asked me all the same questions that I had just answered on paper. Still, he was much better at this than my first caseworker had been. This time, I was able to tell him my story without a whole bunch of intrusive and unsettling questions. He just listened, asked me simple questions when he needed to know more, and otherwise just let me talk at my own pace.

There is one thing about me that really gets the mental health people going. I am normally a very animated guy. Some would even say that I'm twitchy. I just seem to have a lot of energy to spare, and that energy needs somewhere to go. Even when I'm sitting still, I tend to fidget a lot. I am that annoying person who sits at my desk, clicking my pen every two seconds. I have had friends come over and put their hands on my arms, just to stop me from waving them about. Whenever I am seeing a professional for therapy, I must first explain to them that I was like this way before the trauma, and that it's in no way related. It's part of the normal me. Otherwise they all look at me like they think I am really, really anxious, when in fact I am only the regular amount of anxious (for me). The only way to tell the difference is that, when I am actually nervous, my knees bounce up and down. That's my tell.

Once our appointment was over, he sent his report to NATH. This took a couple of weeks, so I was still sitting at home waiting. He agreed that my symptoms were consistent with PTSD. Finally, I was able to access some treatment and begin the healing process. This was the first time in over three months that I felt like I could breathe.

I really liked the psychologist. He had a really easy manner about him, like he would be easy to confide in. I even enquired about seeing him for further treatment. Unfortunately, that's not allowed. Treating me for PTSD when he is the one evaluating my condition for NATH was considered a conflict of interest. That makes sense. Still, one of the hardest things about going to therapy (yes, I had been in therapy before this) is finding a therapist that I feel comfortable working with. If there isn't a connection, trust cannot develop, and therapy just doesn't work under those circumstances.

· · ·

One final thing that I should probably mention. At around this time, my wife and I finally got a divorce. It may seem irrelevant, but it does have some bearing on the situation. You see, the divorce was my idea, but I had agreed to put it off until she had found herself a job. Because of how long she had been away from nursing, she had to meet certain criteria. This necessitated several trips into the big city. Those did not mesh well with the anxiety, let me tell you. I am surprised that I managed to drive us both back and forth without killing us, I was so nervous.

It took almost nine months for her to find a job. Now remember, I had already been supporting her fully for ten years by this point. Well, as soon as she had gotten herself a job, suddenly we could not get those papers signed fast enough. Here I am, with no way of supporting myself and no idea when I might be getting any money. Not to mention the fact that my entire world had just been turned upside down. All I wanted was some time to get my life sorted out. At that point, I was the one needing help. Instead of understanding, I got, "Thanks for everything. Now get out."

THIS IS THE CHAPTER WHERE I CAN FINALLY AFFORD TO EAT AGAIN

F inally, my first check arrived. Suddenly, I was able to afford all those luxuries again, like eating. Oh, and let's not forget the gas.

Because of my recent divorce, and the subsequent rush to get me out the door, one of the first things I had to do was go house hunting. Let me just say that looking for a place to live while suffering from high anxiety is not a pleasant experience. I found a prefect apartment fairly quickly, but my application was not accepted. One rejection was all it took to shut me down for two days. My brain simply couldn't handle it. I was obsessing, thinking that I would never find a place in time. This, despite the fact that I still had almost a month to continue looking. There was absolutely no logic to this feeling, but that's what depression and anxiety do. Because of this, I called the search off, knowing what it was doing to my emotional well-being. Instead, I went back to an apartment complex that I had previously lived in. There, I pretty much begged the manager for an apartment. She agreed, so at least that was settled. It's a nice place, by the way, and cheap.

Almost right away, NATH assigned an occupational therapist to my case. His job was to oversee my progress and to act as a contact for all the people involved in my case. He was the organizer. I really liked him. He always took time to listen to my thoughts and to give me direction. At times, he would come right to my apartment so that we could strategize. He made sure that I was getting to see the right people in order to continue making progress. He also pushed me so that I didn't stagnate. That would have been so easy to do, given my frame of mind at that point. All my brain wanted to do was stay inside and mope. I much preferred talking to him in person, however. He had a very thick accent, and sometimes I wasn't entirely sure what he was saying when we talked on the phone. I must have driven him crazy, asking him to constantly repeat everything. In person, I always understood what he was saying just fine.

Our first task was to come up with a concrete plan for getting me back to work. This required some collaboration between the various parties involved (my employer, NATH, the union), which was the occupational therapist's primary role.

One thing that aggravated me was that he always seemed in a bit of a rush. I realize that it wasn't entirely his fault, though. I know that NATH was putting the pressure on. Sometimes, it seemed as if no one really cared whether I was actually getting better or not, as long as I returned to work as quickly as possible. It was extremely frustrating to feel pushed when I was still hurting so much. Even more so because they had no problem taking their own sweet time when it was me doing the waiting. As I'm sure you will understand, I had a vested interest in making sure that my treatment was successful, rather than just quick. That meant taking the time to do things properly.

Now, I know what you are thinking. Taxpayer dollars and all. I know, I get it. Here's the thing though. I was hurt on the job, serving the public good. I didn't ask for this to happen to me. I figure that I had earned that treatment. I really don't believe that I am asking for too much. I want to get better. I want to go back to my job, or at least *a* job. However, rushing things and failing isn't in anyone's best interest. It just prolongs the entire ordeal because it creates even more trauma. Also, failing again is only going to increase the depression. I started to feel that I was deficient because I couldn't keep up with the official timeline. I'm not a psychology expert, but I still know that making me feel worse about myself probably wasn't a winning strategy.

Anyway, I felt that I had to really dig my heels in with the occupational therapist from time to time. Like, "Whoa there. Let's not get ahead of ourselves." He was telling me the plan for step eight and I was still on step three. Still, most of the time, I felt that he was very helpful. Often, when I did say "whoa," he made sure that my reasons were heard by the case manager.

I was also set up with a personal trainer. Apparently, exercise is good for depression and anxiety, so I am told. I am still not entirely certain that I believe them, but they insisted. As a result, three times a week I was off to the gym. If you knew me, you would know just how funny that is. I don't really do healthy, and I had certainly not been to a gym in years. Probably not since high school.

In my youth, I had been one of those annoying skinny people who could eat all the crap I wanted and never gain a pound. As I aged, my metabolism slowed down. Unfortunately, my appetite did not. I *may* have put on a few extra pounds in the last ten years. I did walk a lot, as I have already said, but only because I had to. Trust me, if I could have rolled my chair around the emergency department, I would have. Getting around at work was as far as I went with exercising. And when I say that I would always eat crap, I mean crap. If the label didn't say Hostess or Coca-Cola, I wouldn't touch it. Sometimes, I would bring a salad in for lunch, just to see the expression on everyone's face. To this day, I still believe that carrot cake is part of a fascist plot. Seriously, what kind of a sick mind would hide vegetables in cake?

I remember one incident when I was at work and a code blue was called on the pediatric ward. That is the call none of us ever want to hear. Most of the time, the ICU nurses go to codes within the hospital. However, they *do not* do kids, so the ER nurses respond to those calls. Anyway, off we ran, up several flights of stairs. When we arrived on the pediatric ward, it turned out to be a false alarm. That was really lucky for me because I would have been no help to anyone at that point. One of my co-workers thought that I was going to go into cardiac arrest myself, right there by the nurses' desk. I was puffing and panting as if I had just run a marathon.

Just to give you an idea of how out of character it is for me to exercise, I will tell you another story. When I first started going to the gym, I posted a picture online of me on an exercise bike. It was during one of my first sessions. I am quite sure that several people at work dropped dead from shock. There were many, many jokes made at my expense that day. I have all your names, and I will have my revenge.

My trainer was really good (I know, I say that about everyone). She was motivating, but not pushy, if you know what I mean. Sometimes my energy would be low, so we would just stick to the simpler exercises. She had me working on the weights, doing stretches, and spending time on the bike. I will admit that I absolutely despise the bike. That is not because I find it difficult. It's just so boring. I essentially have to sit there and peddle for twenty minutes, staring at the wall. I told you, I don't do sitting well. They have a TV overhead, but the sound is turned off, so even that isn't engaging. I'm not one of the world's most disciplined people when it comes to activities I'm not interested in, so peddling the damn bike can seem like a real chore at times.

On occasion, we would have to go outside. I also don't do crowds that well these days, and sometimes the gym would be packed. This was common if we went later in the day. Other times, there would be someone working out that would trigger me. One day, for instance, there was a very elderly gentleman exercising there. I don't know why, but I just kept imagining that he was going to die right in front of us. Then I would have to try to save him. Just the thought of that was enough to make me very nervous. There was a track out back, so we would do my work out there instead, on those occasions when we had to leave. She would have me run up and down the stairs, or we would do some stretches and endurance exercises. The thing I liked best about her was that I never had to explain why. I would just say no, and we would find something else to do instead. She seemed to be the only person who just took me at my word during those early days.

Mainly, we focused on exercises that would be useful once I went back to work. A lot of pushing and pulling, like what I would be expected to do with patients. The whole idea was to keep me in shape, so I didn't go soft. Once my brain was fixed, I still had to be able to do the physical work.

What is especially ironic about this story is that I still go to the gym. My time with the trainer came to an end almost a year ago. However, I have since found that I actually enjoy my time there. Ok, maybe not the bike. In fact, on the occasions that I don't go, it's usually because I don't want to ride the bike. In order to overcome this, I now have a bike at home that I bought secondhand. At least now I can watch my own shows while I peddle. It is much easier to remain disciplined when I only have to do the weights when I go to the gym. I will admit that I have been slacking a little lately, but only because I have been spending so much of my time writing. I get in the zone and don't realize how much time has passed. Suddenly, it's too late in the day to go. See, it's actually *your* fault!

I should also point out that my diet hasn't changed at all. I still eat way too much sugar. In fact, I probably snack more now than I used to. After dinner, I always seem to have the munchies. Apparently, this is a common side effect of some antidepressants. I was quite surprised when I found out about that. It certainly explained a lot, like why I only seem to get hungry in the evenings. So, despite a year and a half of rigorous exercise, I still have the same gut I had when I started. If it weren't for my eating habits, I would be totally ripped I tell you.

Back when all of this first started, I happened upon a kayak that was on sale. Well, my first check from NATH had just come in, so I thought, "why not?" I had rented kayaks a few times in the past and had really enjoyed kayaking. Now, I had one of my very own, so no more excuses. At first, paddling was very hard, and I would tire out rather quickly. Going to the gym definitely helped, as did taking the kayak out consistently. I have developed a lot more strength in my shoulders, so paddling is much easier now. These days, it is one of my favorite things to do. I go out for short paddles as often as I can. Last year I took a three-day trip with my sister. She enjoyed it so much that she bought a kayak as well.

This year, I decided to up the game and bought myself a used sea kayak, the really long ones with the rudder at the back. What I didn't know was that these come in different sizes, apparently. When I tried to take it out for a spin, I found that I was too tall to get into the damn thing. The cockpit was too narrow. Once I had managed to stuff myself in there (which involved moves that would make a contortionist proud), I found that getting out was even worse because I could not bend my knees. My leg got stuck halfway out, and the whole thing tipped into the water. I did a face-plant right into the mud on the shoreline. If you know of anyone that would like a used sea kayak cheap, let me know.

Next year, I hope to try again with a new sea kayak. I will try it out first, this time, before I buy it. My plan is to take it on an extended trip somewhere. Maybe for an entire week. If you know of anyone that is *selling* a used sea kayak cheap, let me know.

...

Of course, the most important development during this time was that I was finally able to get in for some therapy. They sent me to someone who specializes in emotional trauma as well as post-traumatic stress, and I began seeing him once a week. I was so glad, not just because I was finally going to get some treatment, but because they had also found me a good therapist. I did mention how important that is to recovery. If I hadn't liked him, I would have had to continue looking. I don't think that NATH would have given me many other options either.

To begin with, NATH wanted me to attend a special program of their own design. They had developed it specifically for people with PTSD. Unfortunately, this would have involved spending several weeks in another city, as they only offer it in one place. They also offered to put me up in a hotel for the duration of the course. Now, I am sure that their program was designed with only the best of intentions. Also, who doesn't enjoy a trip to the big city (except for me, which we have already established), especially when it involves a stay in a fancy hotel for a few weeks.

As soon as my caseworker suggested this program, I knew that it wasn't for me. I am not sure why they thought that taking me to a strange city, away from all my support systems, was a good idea. Any progress that I made while in the program would have been immediately undone by the level of anxiety and loneliness I would have experienced just being there. Also, considering how clueless they had appeared to be when it came to PTSD, I wasn't exactly certain that I wanted to put my care into their hands. When I had first reached out to them, they didn't even appear to have a grasp on what PTSD was. Up until that point, our relationship had not exactly been built on a foundation of trust. My caseworker was a little put out when I declined the offer, to her it must have seemed as though I was saying that I didn't really want to get better.

"Well, we do have an alternative," she said, as if it was by far the inferior option. "We can set you up with a therapist right in your city." Her tone suggested that I was on a game show and had just been offered the consolation prize. From my point of view, this seemed to be the superior option by far. Staying at home was pretty much a no-brainer.

There are many types of treatment for PTSD, but the one used by my therapist is something called EMDR. It stands for Eye Movement

Desensitization and Reprocessing. Apparently, it's a relatively new type of therapy and has been getting very good results. The whole concept is based on the process that occurs in the brain during REM sleep. When we dream, our brains are busy sorting through the events of the day and storing those events into our long-term memories. If you've watched the movie *50 First Dates*, you'll know what I'm talking about. As you may recall, the entire basis of PTSD is that memories get "stuck" in short-term memory instead of being processed. EMDR is used to trick the brain into thinking that the patient is in REM sleep, so that it can process and store those memories the way it should. In essence, those memories (hopefully) get moved into long-term memory, so that the brain is not reliving the same moment over and over again. As a result, the patient is able to move forward. When it was first developed, the practitioner would sit before the patient and move an object, such as a pen, back and forth before the patient's eyes. Hence the name. As the practice evolved, it was found that other repetitive movements could have the same effect.

When I first went to see my therapist, I was expecting the traditional appointments. You know, lie on a couch and talk about my feelings. Tell him about my childhood. That sort of thing. Instead, with EMDR, you don't talk at all. It was bizarre, sitting there in silence. Not what I had been imagining at all. I really had my doubts at first because the whole thing just felt rather weird. I would sit there and think about all the events that were troubling me. My hands were in front of me, resting on a table with palms down. As I combed through my memories, he would sit opposite me and just tap lightly on the back of my hands. Sounds totally hokey, I know. The thing is it really does work. At least, it worked for me.

In fact, it worked so well that I was already feeling much better after only a few sessions. My anxiety was subsiding and my mood improved substantially. At that point, I don't believe I had been able to experience happiness in months. Suddenly, I had joy back in my life again. It wasn't all the time. The treatments didn't work that fast, after all. It was certainly more than never, though, which was a very welcome change.

Not that there weren't setbacks along the way. In one of the sessions, I was thinking about the young child that we had treated. Suddenly, an ambulance picked that exact second to blare its siren, right outside the window. My therapist had to peel me off the ceiling. It shocked me, but I thought I would get over it without too much difficulty. Boy, was I mistaken. After leaving his office, I wandered around the neighborhood for a while. His office is located just around the corner from an area with several artsy little shops. I was standing in the middle of one of the stores when everything hit me. I started to experience some very disturbing thoughts and flashbacks of that day. I quickly retreated to my car and drove away, which was probably not the best plan given how upset I was. I'm certain my driving skills were somewhat erratic, so it is very fortunate that I made it home safely. Once inside, I ended up spending another day curled up in a ball on the floor. Still, despite a few such episodes, a great deal of progress was made in a reasonably short period of time.

The most surprising detail that I discovered during my treatments was that the cause of my breakdown was not what I had originally thought it to be. The natural assumption would be that my PTSD was caused by all the horrible events I had witnessed during that day. That is what I believed, anyway. However, as I went over the memories of that day in my mind, I found that the event that disturbed me the most did not involve a patient at all. Instead, it was the moment that Duine Gearr had started to cry. She had spent the entire day working her butt off because no one had been there to help her. I had spent the whole day taking the sickest patients because no one else was able to manage. In that instant, I think that I experienced a moment of perfect empathy. I understood her frustration on such an intimate level that it essentially became like a spike, driving in to my subconscious. Despite all the stress of that day, those experiences were not at the root of my trauma at all. They had most certainly added to it, of course. After all, who would not find those events to be traumatizing. Still, I would have been able to look at those events with a certain level of detachment, as I had always done in the past. However, when I saw pain and anger in the eyes of someone I knew and cared about, it was a different story altogether. Especially as I identified so strongly with her in that moment. Because of this, I couldn't remain detached. That was the event that I couldn't let go of. It was a huge revelation.

There is a terrible irony to this. It is my empathy that made me a great nurse. It is also at the very heart of my eventual breakdown.

Anyone else who has ever had a significant epiphany like that will under-stand when I say what an enormous relief it was to me. It was like having a huge weight lifted from my shoulders. I felt unburdened and about a thou-sand pounds lighter. That was probably the most cathartic moment of my entire life, up until that point. Being able to recognize and process that event was an enormous step in my recovery. Not to give you the impression that I was suddenly somehow magically cured. I still had a great deal of work to do. After all, we're talking about fourteen years of piled up events that I had stuffed down and never dealt with. No one moves past all of that in one go. Still, it was a very significant breakthrough for me. I described it to my thera-pist as carrying a truck in one hand and several bricks in another. The bricks were still there, but the truck was now gone. Bricks, all by themselves, are much easier to carry.

I was also taught some pretty good coping skills for when I felt my anxiety rising. One method that I started to use is called tapping. I just tap lightly, right below the kneecaps and it helps to calm me down. I have no idea why, but I find it to be very soothing. This method has helped me to get through some of my worst episodes.

My home environment is also very important. I have put in a great deal of effort making it a space that I can feel secure in. The décor is cozy, and I have littered the place with art and various other items that relax me. (I collect dragon figurines. Nerdy I know.) Nothing fancy, mind you. All the art is cheap. Some of it is even a little creepy, but that's my style. I also have a lot of framed photographs. Some are of old friends. Others are of locations that are important to me. I have a few photos that my sister took, and they are spectacular.

One photo is particularly special. When I was younger, I would often travel deep into the bush with some friends of mine. I even helped to build many of the trails through this area. Whenever we would go there, I had a camping spot that was absolutely breathtaking. It became my spot. One day, a friend suggested that when I start to feel anxious, I should go to my happy place. So, I did. I am quite certain that she meant figuratively, but I didn't care. I drove down to the area, almost destroying the undercarriage of my car in the process. Apparently, my car doesn't like off-roading. I then hiked into the bush for the day. While there, I took a picture of my little spot. Now, I can see it whenever I want.

The smell of my apartment is also very important. I don't know why, but I have always found the smell of vanilla to be particularly effective at calming me down. I bought a contraption that looks rather like a fondue set. You place some scented wax on top, and the smell of vanilla is released as the wax melts down. It fills the entire apartment with the aroma. Unfortunately, I had to turn it off a few weeks ago. Having it on all the time means that I have gotten so used to the smell that I can't even tell it's there anymore.

For getting to sleep, I have managed to devise a little trick. You see, falling asleep is the hardest part for me. As soon as my head hits that pillow, my brain will suddenly wake up and want to party. My brain is kind of an asshole that way. All the insomniacs out there will know exactly what I am talking about. My mind is like that annoying party guest that won't leave your house till three in the morning, despite the fact that everyone else went home hours ago. There's me, ready for dreamland, and my brain pops up with, "Hey, what about this global warming?" Then I'm lying there for hours staring at the ceiling, wishing that I could somehow manage to smother myself with a pillow.

Recently, I have figured out a great way to keep those random thoughts away. When I lie down and get relaxed, I make up little speeches in my head. Sounds insane, but it is actually very effective. Usually, it's something about history (nerd), or some other topic that I know a lot about. I pretend that I am giving someone a lesson on some fascinating historical event, and it keeps those stray ideas from getting into my brain. Essentially, it helps me to focus on one thing at a time, so that the extraneous thoughts are kept mostly at bay. I might just be the only person ever to bore *myself* to sleep.

. . .

One thing that I have found hard to accept is just how easily I was replaced at work. I've always thought of myself as being very good at my job. I really thought that I was an integral part of the team there. I'm also pretty smart, and I have a great deal of knowledge rattling around in my head. There are fourteen years of experience in there, after all. I think I still have a great deal to offer. However, once I had left, the department moved on without even a pause. Barely anyone even seemed to notice. That's a pretty depressing real-ization. I thought that I was important, that I mattered. Instead it was, "So sorry for your troubles. Don't let the door hit you on the way out." I wasn't expecting the ER to grind to a halt, just because I wasn't around anymore. I am confident, not arrogant. It would have been nice, however, if I had detected even a small sense of loss from the people who remained.

Part of that feeling probably comes from the fact that there are so many new people there now. It's only been a year and a half, but I walk through the department these days and I only recognize a third of the people. It's hard to miss what they never knew. Still, at least part of that feeling comes from not being valued for the work that we do. The message is that we are all easily replaceable, and that lack of appreciation falls squarely on management.

A few months ago, I was visiting the department. One of my former co-workers approached me and called me aside. She told me that she thought my leaving was a real loss to the ER. She also told me how much she had appreciated working with me when we were both still there. I almost broke down in tears right in the middle of the hallway we were standing in. That was the first (and last) time anyone had said those words to me.

WHAT COULD POSSIBLY
GO WRONG?

After several months of therapy, I was deemed fit to go back to work. I was not cured by any stretch of the imagination. I was still experiencing a great deal of anxiety most of the time. I often had bouts of depression as well. Still, I had made a lot of progress, and my symptoms had certainly become more manageable than they had been only a few months before. When I did feel anxious, I had several methods to calm myself down.

Unfortunately, NATH has this rather stupid and unfortunate rule. When an employee goes back to work, that employee can only return to their former position. Again, emotional trauma is still a fairly new concept. As a result, the rules haven't quite caught up. If I had suffered a physical injury, putting me back into my old job would make perfect sense. In such a circumstance, why would I not return to the ER. Having PTSD, however, is something quite different. In those with post-traumatic stress, it is not the reality of the environment that is hazardous, it is the perception of the environment. In other words, I don't need to be safe; I need to *feel* safe. Putting me right back into the environment that had caused my breakdown was setting me up for failure. Any new experiences simply reinforced the initial trauma.

Just as with my previous back injury, I was sent back on a graduated return-to-work plan. I think that during the first week, I was only there for eight-hour shifts. I also wasn't taking any patients of my own. I was just there to help out where I could. The whole idea was to gently ease me back in.

On my very first day back, one of our nurses had a patient who was not doing very well. In fact, he was dying. He had a do-not-resuscitate order in place, so the plan was to keep him as comfortable as possible. He was concerned, however, because his entire family was flying in and he wanted a chance to say goodbye to all of them. This necessitated a slight change in our treatment plan. Essentially, we were not trying to save him, but we were working quite hard to keep him going. We wanted him to remain alive long enough for everyone to get there. The department was very busy that day, so the only people that were available to help the nurse were me and one of our managers (who doesn't usually deal directly with patients). Together, the three of us worked to prolong his life just a little bit longer.

Despite the urgency of our work, I was actually handling it quite well. I did feel anxious, because that never fully goes away, but I wasn't feeling excessively stressed or anything. Perhaps that's because I knew the situation wasn't life or death. If he had passed away during this time, we would not have intervened at all. I also knew that he wasn't my patient, so I didn't feel that burden of responsibility. That took the pressure off, I believe.

Of course, that's when the trouble started. It seems that the day before my return, there had been a bad trauma. Naturally, this meant that everyone was talking about it all day long. The three of us had taken our patient out of the department for a CT scan, and the nurse and manager started to discuss the previous day's events in vivid detail. Listening to this, my anxiety level just shot right through the roof. The story was too much, it cut too deep. I was unable to keep myself calm, and I basically ran from the room. I ended up sitting in one of the staircases for about half an hour, hugging my knees to my chin.

Anxiety is a little like physical pain. At least, that has been my experience. Pain is much easier to control when it is maintained at a low level. That is why we always tell patients to take medication when the pain level starts to rise, rather than waiting for it to get bad. Once pain reaches a certain level, it becomes very hard to bring it back down again. Similarly, I can control my anxiety when it is low. However, once it becomes a full-blown panic attack, none of my calming techniques work anymore. Only time and a non-stimulating environment will bring my stress back down to a manageable level. Thankfully, the stairwell I was sitting in is rarely used, so I had the space to myself. In time, the panic receded.

Before I could even think about going back, though, I needed something to bring my anxiety down further. I wasn't quite back to baseline yet. I had forgotten my anxiety medication at home, so I went to the med room and grabbed one from our stock. I think it took another half hour before I was actually ready to return to work. For the rest of the shift, I would basically run away from anyone who even attempted to discuss the previous day. Because it had been such a big event, that meant moving around a lot!

The gentleman we had been caring for made it, by the way. I think he finally passed away a few days later, with his entire family in attendance. Death is never good, but those always seem like the best deaths to me.

One of the things I am now very strict on is debriefs after every critical incident. This was no exception. Even though it wasn't technically a "critical" incident, it had still been physically and emotionally taxing. For that reason, I demanded that we still needed to have one. The next day, I grabbed the other two nurses and herded them into an empty room so that we could talk. It was short and sweet. Basically, we all felt good about the way things had transpired. We had done everything correctly, and the outcome had been a positive one. Still, how do we know that unless we check in with each other. Again, it's that divide between the physical and the emotional. Just because it was my perception that everything had gone well, that doesn't mean that everyone involved had felt the same way. This is why we check in. This is why debriefs are so essential.

A few days later, I was in the med room with a co-worker. I saw her take out the same medication I had taken, only for a patient this time. Then she recorded it in one of our med books. This was new to me. Before I had gone off work, we had never recorded these medications individually. Instead, we would only count them at the end of each day. We had never signed out single doses like that. This differs from our narcotics, where every single dose must be accounted for. I happened to mention to my co-worker that I had probably screwed up the count a few days ago because I had not known this. I said it very casually, because at the time I didn't think anything of it. Well, that really blew up in my face.

My co-worker was completely taken aback by the fact that I had taken a medication for myself in this manner. In my own mind, I didn't really see what the problem was. We will often take things like Tylenol when we have a headache at work. Not many of us would even think twice about that. I was also on the medication at home, and I had simply forgotten to bring it with me. In the end though, I hadn't really stopped to consider what I was actually doing. My brain wasn't working on all gears because, at the time, I had been so anxious. Really, what I had taken wasn't just any medication. It was a controlled medication, and they are controlled for a reason. In retrospect, I never should have done that.

The worst part was that, because of my disclosure, I had totally wigged out my co-worker. I had put her in a very awkward position, and she ended up having to report the incident to the manager. Then she ended up carrying around all this guilt for having had to "rat me out." In reality, I wasn't upset with her at all. I felt just awful for having put her in that position to begin with. It had been completely unfair of me. A few days later, I managed to catch up to her, and I apologized profusely.

My manager was pretty cool about it. I think she saw the entire incident as inevitable. She had thought, right from the beginning, that it was stupid to put me right back into the ER. It was an environment that was bound to increase my anxiety level. She blamed NATH for putting me in this situation in the first place.

For the rest of my graduated return, things did not go well. After that first day, my anxiety stayed at a constantly elevated level while I was at work. I just wasn't able to relax again, after that. Everything seemed to bother me, especially the noise level. The entire department was one big trigger, all the time. I found that I could only work in the monitored area during the mornings because, as it became busier toward the afternoon, the noise level would reach an unmanageable level for me. I couldn't even contemplate taking a patient assignment. I was far too wound up all the time. For the entire four weeks, I basically wandered around the department, starting IVs and trying to keep myself busy with small tasks.

I also spent a great deal of time hiding out in one of the quiet rooms. This didn't help my state of mind. In fact, it made me feel worse. Now, I was also worried that my co-workers would think I was lazy. In reality, anxiety takes a heavy toll all its own. All my energy was being consumed just trying to hold myself together until the end of the shift. After that, I had nothing left to share. Still, I felt as though I was letting everyone down.

I was also suffering the same lapses in concentration that I had experienced the first time around. I continuously forgot things that should have been second nature to me by now. I couldn't make decisions. Basically, I didn't feel that I could do anything right. I don't mean that in a bad way. I knew it wasn't because I was stupid. It was just a symptom of my condition. The reason I felt bad about it is that those lapses can put patients at risk. If I neglected to do something critical, I could end up causing serious harm, even death. I would never be able to live with that.

There was a positive side to this experience. I think that month was the only time during my entire ordeal that I managed to sleep without any difficulty. When I would get home after my shift, I was so tired that I basically collapsed into bed. Glass half full, right?

On one particular day, I happened to be helping out in the ambulatory area. At some point, we had a patient arrive in cardiac arrest. Now, what you have to understand is that everyone who works in an emergency room does so because we are trauma junkies (I even have a shirt that says "trauma junkie" on it). This often means that when a critical patient is brought in, the entire department suddenly empties of staff. All the doctors, all the nurses, everyone wants to get in on the action. At this time, there was a patient in ambulatory who was in quite a lot of pain. I wanted to get him something to make him more comfortable, but to do that I needed a doctor's order. I do not exaggerate when I tell you that there was not a single doctor to be found, anywhere. Every single one of them had gone rushing into the trauma room. Of course, if I wanted to get that order, I would have to go in there myself. That was a prospect I was not looking forward to. When I walked in, I saw one of the other nurses doing CPR. She looked right at me and asked if I would take over for her. I jumped, made a little squeaking noise, shook my head, and ran out the door. Someone else ended up having to get the order. Another of my co-workers thought the entire episode was hilarious. Me, not so much.

There was another event that really illustrated how much had changed in the department. At this point, I had only been gone for seven months or so. I was helping out, as usual, when a patient was brought in with chest pain. I told the nurse who was working there that I would help him. I entered the room first and was busy getting the patient hooked up to the monitor. This is when the other nurse came in. He was fairly new to our department, so he didn't really know who I was. Because of this, he proceeded to show me how to properly put the patient on the monitor. He went through the entire procedure, step-by-step. In fairness, he was doing an excellent job of teaching me. Unfortunately, after all those years in the ER, I had no need for his instructions. I must have had some sort of perturbed look on my face because he stopped suddenly and didn't say another word to me.

It was during this time that I did something spectacularly dumb. There was a job up for grabs that I really wanted. I had gone for an interview and felt that I had done quite well. I really thought that I had a good shot at it. Unfortunately, because of the stupid rules again, I had to finish the GRTW before I could accept the new position. This was not an easy thing to accomplish, as I was obviously failing quite spectacularly. I was set on getting that new position, though. I talked to my occupational therapist about it, and we conspired to keep my difficulties under wraps for the time being. I just needed to get through the process so that I could move on. In hindsight, this was a very bad idea.

I didn't end up getting the job. I was told that I had given the best interview out of all the people they had seen. In the end, however, they had chosen to go with someone more experienced in that area. I was devastated, of course. I had been so sure I was going to get the position. As a result, I had put all my eggs into one basket, based on that assumption. Essentially, it was painfully obvious that I could not continue to work in the ER. My return to work had been a complete failure, as I had not managed to carry out any of the duties that would be expected of me. During the entire month, I had not even been capable of taking a patient of my own. Having me manage an entire team was simply out of the question. Unfortunately, the only ones who knew this were me and my occupational therapist. We had deliberately kept this information from NATH, based on the premise that I was going to get that other job. Now we had to go to them, looking rather foolish, and tell them what had actually transpired. They were not pleased and more than a little confused by the whole matter. In the end, however, they had no choice but to continue my claim. If it hadn't worked, it hadn't worked, even though we had lied about it. I was off work once again.

Another positive thing did come out of my time being back at work. My family doctor had sent me to see a psychiatrist to go over my medications. She had prescribed an antidepressant for me, but she wasn't as confident with her choice as she would have liked to be. It wasn't her area of expertise, and there are several other medications I could have been taking instead. Plus, many antidepressants have some pretty unpleasant side effects, especially since I had recently begun a new relationship. I was really hoping to change to something different.

Of course, after my doctor gave me the referral, it took several months to even get a call back. Eventually, I was given an appointment to see the psychiatrist on call at the local mental health clinic. When I arrived that day, I was full of expectations. Unfortunately, the guy I eventually saw appeared to be totally disinterested. Bored, even. To tell you the truth, he gave me the impression that he was one of those people who was inches away from retiring. You know what I mean, right? Like his brain was already on a beach somewhere, sipping margaritas, and everything else was just a distraction. He didn't change a damn thing and sent me on my way.

Lucky for me, I still worked in the ER. I told you that membership has its privileges. Even better, we had a psych area just down the hall. I even knew most of the psychiatrists who worked there. Since I was in the department anyway, working, I asked the nurses down there if they could squeeze me in for a few minutes. They agreed, and the psychiatrist that I saw changed all my medications for me. She upped my dosage on one and changed another to one with fewer side effects. According to her, the reason that I was having so much difficulty was that I was way undermedicated. After making the switches, my mood was somewhat more stable.

A LITTLE MORE HELPFUL

After the graduated return had failed, I was referred back to the original psychologist for another assessment—the same one that had performed the first assessment. Of course, it took another couple of months to get a new appointment. NATH was in standby mode, so all I could do was wait as well. Once again, I had to get used to sitting at home with nothing to do. At least watching TV was getting a little easier for me. I still couldn't watch any medical shows, though.

When I finally did manage to get in to see the psychologist for the second appointment, we had to go through the entire process all over again. I had to sit in my little room, filling out the three million questionnaires until my thumb was ready to fall off. Yes, I was still depressed. No, I wasn't suicidal. Then, we sat in his office and chatted again. This time around, he diagnosed me with a generalized anxiety disorder. As a result, it was agreed upon that I could not return to the ER for work.

After receiving this diagnosis, the entire process had to be changed. My condition was now considered to be a "permanent disability," and that meant I was no longer eligible for NATH benefits. Luckily, this doesn't mean that I was kicked to the curb. In true bureaucratic fashion, they simply moved me over to a whole new section of NATH called ALMH. I think it's a little like having my kitchen located in an entirely different apartment. Essentially, their purpose was to find me a new job that wouldn't end up freaking me out every day. I was also given a new caseworker.

I must admit, I was not pleased with the whole permanent disability idea. I like to think that someday I will be back to my old normal. As you may have gathered, I am not exactly fond of the whole anxiety experience. I would take it back for a full refund, if I could. Still, if it is to be permanent, I suppose it's nice to have the label there. It means that I have some protection as I go forward, since it will most likely impact me wherever I end up.

Through ALMH, I also ended up receiving less money per month. For some reason, the bean counters over there figure that the worse your condition gets, the less you need their financial support. I can confidently tell you that this is not actually the case. In reality, my expenses have gone up. Though my medication costs are *mostly* covered, I still have to pay some money out of my own pocket. If I want to keep up with my exercise, something that NATH definitely wants me to continue, I now have to pay for my own gym membership (it was all free while I had the personal trainer). In addition, I now had to pay my employer for the benefits that I received through our extended medical plan, because they were no longer covered. They also took away my parking pass, which was a real kick in the teeth. Less money, more costs. Makes the usual amount of sense.

Another thing that happened, once I was deemed to have a permanent injury, is that NATH granted me a disability award. Sounds great, doesn't it? Finally, an acknowledgment of the emotional pain and suffering that I have had to endure because I was injured on the job. Of course, there's always a catch with these people. All the money that I was awarded came right off my NATH benefits. Apparently, if they didn't do this, it would be "double dipping." In other words, I got bupkus. "We're so sorry for all that has happened to you. Here is some compensation to make things easier. Oh, but wait, you can only look at it. It's not actually for you." If I had managed to find another job by that point, the money would have been mine. Instead, I get compensation for not being able to work, then I get penalized for not being able to work. Such is the logic of NATH.

I also get a separate check every month now. The permanent disability people also awarded me a small monthly sum. This is sent to me from an entirely new section of NATH. It makes me wonder how many sections they have hidden away over there. Are they connected? Are they allowed to talk to one another? Do they have to wear different colored uniforms to identify themselves? These are the things that I would like to know. The check itself is not very much money. Apparently, I will continue to receive it until I retire. Of course, this is dutifully deducted from my regular monthly benefits as well. They also put a small percentage of these funds into an RRSP every month. At my age, when I retire I should have just enough in there to buy myself a new pair of pants. Depending, of course, on inflation. I have made plans to treat myself.

At this point, someone decided that I didn't even have PTSD. I still have all the symptoms, but now it was referred to as a "workplace stress injury." If it walks like a duck and talks like a duck, let's call it an elephant and hope that no one notices. I get suspicious when things like this happen. In fact, it makes me feel very angry. It is like my condition is being minimized somehow. By being relabeled, someone in an office somewhere can now say, "Look, we don't have a PTSD problem." It's also as if someone is trying to tell me how I feel inside. Like my emotions are no longer valid, because I supposedly have this "other" condition. "Oh, you can't have hypervigilance. That's a symptom of post-traumatic stress." This is probably me just being a little paranoid, but it still stung a great deal. I should clarify that there is such a thing as a workplace stress injury, but there are differences. As far as I can gather, a workplace stress injury is more specific to one single event, and it also tends to be short lived. Some of the symptoms of PTSD may be present, but not enough to meet the threshold for a PTSD diagnosis. I hope that I got the definition right.

There was another absurdity that came up during this time. I was reamed out by my employer for attempting to organize an online survey. I had done this in an attempt to learn just how many of my fellow nurses were also suffering. In my mind, I believed that the first step in creating a solution would be to get a better idea of how widespread the problem was. For the survey, I used a standardized set of questions that were designed specifically for PTSD. The questions asked nurses to rate their feelings of stress in various situations on a scale of one to ten. I put up notices around the hospital and got several responses almost immediately. This is when someone with authority freaked out. I was told that I was conducting an unauthorized study and that I had to desist immediately. There was concern that all the nurses would now think that they had PTSD, despite the fact that I had stated this was not the case right in the opening statement of the questionnaire. I wrote, very plainly, "Answering yes to any of these questions does not indicate that you have post-traumatic stress. It only indicates that you have some of the symptoms and may be at greater risk. If any concerns do come up for you while you are answering these questions, make sure that you consult with a mental health professional right away." Apparently, that wasn't clear enough for them, and I had to take the survey down.

Because the survey had been up for such a short time, I wasn't even able to use the responses that I had already received. They would have created a bias, greatly skewing the results. Of course, the people who felt most strongly on the issue were the first to respond and had the highest test scores as a result. It hadn't been up long enough to gather data from those who were not as stressed. I can remember that 90 percent of the people who did take the survey were somewhere on the PTSD scale (people who have some of the symptoms, but do not meet the full criteria for a diagnosis).

During this time, my anxiety had continued unabated. It did decrease a little, but only because I was locked up at home again, where I felt a little safer. Still, I did have my moments. One day, they were testing all the fire alarms in my apartment building. I knew what was happening, yet I still jumped about five feet in the air every time the bell went off. This happened once every couple of minutes, and there are a lot of apartments here. I ended up having to go out because I just couldn't take it anymore.

It was also during this time that I really began to isolate myself. I just didn't feel safe going outside very much. I went to the gym, but I never talked to anyone there. I saw far less of my friends from work. I wasn't able to go by there very often, because just being there was now a trigger for me. My friends, in turn, were busy working all the time.

I did start a new relationship during this period. Fortunately, it was with somebody I already knew or it would never have happened. Not going outside, it's so hard to meet new people. The problem is she happened to be just as anti-social as I was. Now, I had someone to *not* go anywhere with. Still, it was so nice having someone around with whom I could just drop my guard. When I am around most people, as infrequently as that occurs, I always have to put on a front. I have to at least appear as if everything is normal. The reality is that, most of the time, I'm not feeling normal at all. Most of the time I am secretly falling apart inside. With my new girlfriend, I didn't have to put on airs. I could just be my sloppy, neurotic, anxiety-ridden self. It was so amazing to have that level of understanding, even for a little while. I am not going to fill you in on what happened. That story is still a little too personal to share.

To be quite honest, I think that I make a lot of people more than a little uncomfortable. I get the sense that some even go out of their way to avoid me. Part of this stems from the fact that most people don't want to talk about mental health, I am sure. It can be even more discomfiting when it is coming from a man. I have noticed that when women express feelings of sadness, there is usually a lot of support from others. They get all sorts of inspiring messages. Sometimes I envy them for that. For guys, there seems to be an unwritten rule that we should just "suck it up." Emotions are a sign of weakness. Anxiety is especially unmanly because we're not supposed to be afraid, ever. I have been fighting this battle on my own, every day, for almost two years now. I could count on the fingers of one hand the people that have given me any real support. I'm not saying this to make anyone feel guilty. I have managed ok so far. I just want people to be aware of it, so maybe attitudes can start to change. I don't want to be holding it in all the time anymore.

There's also the distinct possibility that I am partly to blame for this situation. I don't always share as much as I should with others. I definitely don't tell many people when I am really hurting. Emotional vulnerability is not exactly my strong suit. Even now, when I know full well the possible consequences of keeping those emotions hidden.

...

Back to the story.

The first time that my new caseworker attempted to contact me, I was asleep and missed her call. I called right back once I woke up, but could only get through to her assistant's voice mail. I did leave a message, but no one got back to me. Next day I called again and left another message. This went on for a week. I was convinced that the assistant was punishing me for not answering the first phone call. I knew she was busy, but the whole not getting back to me for a week thing seemed a little bit suspicious. Surely, somewhere in there she would have had five minutes to spare.

A few other people became involved at that point. One of them worked for my employer, and her role was to help me find a different job. I would still be working as an RN, just not in the ER anymore. We have something called a "duty to accommodate" in our contract. Basically, this means that if I am no longer able to perform my job, they are obligated to find me a job that I can still do. I even get first pick. So if I find a job I want, they have to consider my application before all others. The only thing I could not do was bump someone out of an existing job.

Even this, however, was more complicated than you would think. Of course it was. When I had seen the psychologist, he had made recommendations on what work I could no longer do. He was contracted by NATH, though, so his recommendations could only be related to the original PTSD. Basically, I could not work in the ER or around children anymore. The reasoning, of course, is that these places and people would be triggering for me. Those were the only stipulations he could make. This did not cover me for any difficulties I might have related to the ongoing anxiety I was experiencing. There were several more situations that I could no longer tolerate, but from ALMH's perspective, they didn't matter.

For instance, I knew that any job requiring direct patient care was not going to work for me. On the wards, the pace is certainly different from the ER, but that doesn't mean it's any easier. Sure, you get your assignment of six patients to look after, but then there's the two patients in the hall, two in the TV room, and the guy they have stuffed into the broom closet. It's chaotic and noisy, and all the rooms are very small and cramped. Just as in my old job, no one gets the care they are entitled to. It's simply too busy. This would have led to the same moral distress I had always felt in the ER. I would have lasted about an hour in that environment before I would have gone completely loopy.

Around this time, I had a friend who was admitted to the hospital. Just visiting her for a few hours a day was enough to make me very anxious, and I didn't even have to do anything. I did help them out by starting an IV on my friend (she has tiny veins), but that was it. Again, it was the constant level of noise. There was no way in hell that I was going to tolerate working there.

As it turns out, my employer can impose their own restrictions on where I can work, totally separate from ALMH. For this, I needed to get a doctor's note. Now, my doctor doesn't know what I can and can't do, except for what I inform her of. She did write the letter for me, but I had to tell her what to say in it. This also led to a great deal of confusion, since the two groups of people were often at cross-purposes, due to having two separate criteria for my job search. ALMH would say, "What about this job?" My employer would reply that I wouldn't be able to manage in that position. Back and forth it went.

The person that had been assigned to aid me in my job search did not seem very helpful at first, either. Most of the time, I wasn't even able to contact her. Those rare occasions when I did manage to reach her, she seemed to be totally out of the loop. This is not meant to rag on her, however. The deck was stacked against us both from the very beginning, I believe. She is the sole person responsible for handling every case in our area. I have no idea how many of us there were, but I can state with perfect confidence that it was probably a lot of people. I also possess firsthand experience when it comes to communicating with NATH and ALMH, so I am well aware of the difficulties that she faced in this area. In the end, I had to do most of my own legwork.

I was also trying to find a job that was more behind the scenes. My ideal job would have been as an educator somewhere. I know some stuff. I'm also pretty good at passing that stuff on to others. My second idea was to take a manager's position somewhere. That is still stressful, but it's a different kind of stress, I think. It's definitely less noisy, and I would have had a door I could close when needed.

Once again, the rules got in the way. These are considered to be above my previous job, and so are not covered by the duty to accommodate. I was only eligible for jobs at the same level I was at before—that of a regular RN. The problem, of course, is that most regular RN jobs are on the floors. Because they couldn't help me, I would have to pursue any management jobs on my own. In the meantime, I was getting multiple phone calls from people offering me every inappropriate position that came up.

There was one job that I was very excited about. That is until I found out that a friend of mine was already in the position. Apparently, they had told him to temporarily fill in until someone "better" could be hired. He was pretty pissed about the whole arrangement, and rightly so. He was also an ex ER nurse, and they thought that he was too rough around the edges to hold a management position on a permanent basis. Well, that pretty much counted me out too, then.

I did go to the interview, but I was already having some serious reservations because of what my friend had told me. Then, they were almost an hour late in summoning me. By that point, I had started to believe that I might have gone to the wrong place. I was actually collecting my stuff to leave when they finally called my name. Once I did get in there, the entire process was already doomed. I was tired, hungry, and crabby. I'm sure I gave the worst interview that they had ever seen. I doubt that I answered a single question appropriately. Turns out, they already knew who they wanted for the position anyway, so I hadn't had a chance to begin with. That made me feel a little better about my performance, though it also pissed me off even more than I had been during the interview. I could have shown up completely naked and answered all their questions with interpretive dance and it would not have made any difference. This is quite common in our organization. They already have someone for the position, but they can't just hire that person without going through the entire process, even if that entire process is a complete sham. It's their little way of saying "screw you" to the union, I think. They obey the letter of the contract without paying any mind to the spirit. You can start to understand why that place messed me up so bad.

After that horrible experience, I applied for another position. This was a manager position also, but I would be one of only two nurses (one part-time). In reality, I would only have been the boss of me. Still, the pay is better as a manager. It was a great fit as well, because the job required many of the same skills I had already developed as an ER nurse. As a result, I would already be familiar with most of what the work entailed. I went to the interview with a little more enthusiasm than I had the previous one. I was very excited, and this time I talked up a storm, with my arms waving madly in the air. (I'm Welsh. We do that.) They called me an hour later. "You had the best interview, but we went with someone with more experience." Now where had I heard that before?

While all of this was going on, I was still not getting much help from anyone. I think I was putting more energy into finding a job than I would if I actually *had* a job. It was a lot more stressful as well.

It is a fact, reinforced through first-hand experience, that suffering from a mental illness makes this entire process a great deal more difficult. That is something no one appears to take into account. Again, post-traumatic stress is such a new diagnosis in health care, though it really shouldn't be. Regardless, there is an assumption that the worker can navigate their own way through the system. A person with fully functioning faculties probably could with little difficulty. Increased stress and anxiety strongly impacted my personal ability to do this, however. Every action I took on my own had a price. I would often go an entire day without getting out of bed at all. On those days, I couldn't manage even basic chores. After a while, I passed right through depression and on into despondence. There were many days that I was unable to put any effort into the job search at all. Lucky for me, no one official appeared to notice. That total lack of contact did have its upside.

I even applied for an educator position in another hospital. It had been posted for eight months, so I figured I had a good shot at it. No one else seemed in a rush to claim it anyway. Apparently not! They didn't even call me in for an interview. I did find that common with some of the management-level positions that I applied for. Because of the duty to accommodate, some managers would not even acknowledge my applications. It's as if they thought that, because I was guaranteed a position somewhere, why should they waste a management spot on me. The duty to accommodate appeared to be holding me back at times.

One other position that I applied for was as a diabetes nurse. This job entailed teaching newly diagnosed diabetic patients about nutrition, exercise, etc. Now all ER nurses know a little bit about everything. However, we each have things that we know really well, and things we don't. It's what makes us such a great team. Every person has a piece of the big puzzle, each knowing different things. One of the things I know really well is diabetes. My friends would say that it's because of the way I eat. I am probably one meal away from diabetes myself, most of the time. In reality, it's because I studied up on it extensively. Diabetes fascinates me, probably because it's so complex. It affects so many systems. You might recall that I had even done a case study on it, back when I was doing the ER course. Apparently, though, that wasn't enough. There is a whole separate course that is needed to be a diabetes nurse, so I wasn't even considered. At least my friends got a good laugh at the irony of the whole situation.

It was getting very frustrating. I kept finding jobs and thinking that I would be perfect for each one. Apparently, no one else agreed with me.

Finally, I did find two positions that were both non-management and that I thought I could do without over-stressing myself. One was in a clinic inside the hospital. The other one was in home care. I informed the woman who was supposed to be organizing all this stuff for me, but it was a while before I heard back from her. Once she did contact me, she got in touch with both managers and arranged for some shadowing shifts. Those are shifts where I follow another nurse around for the day so that I can get a feel for the job. The one good thing about a duty to accommodate is that any regular (non-management) job I wanted I could pretty much take. No interviews. I ended up with one day shadowing in the clinic, and two days in home care.

Shadowing is great. Basically, all I have to do is observe. It gives me the opportunity to really experience the job from a neutral perspective. I get to view it from the outside, which removes the stress and anxiety from the equation.

I knew within twenty minutes that I really wanted the clinic job. It was the exact opposite of the ER. It involved meeting with surgical patients and going over all of their information with them. This was done to avoid any surprises on the day of their surgery. They would come in, the nurse would ask them questions, go over any information they needed pre-op, and just generally make sure that everything was ready to go. Occasionally it wasn't, and their OR date would have to be postponed in those cases.

I would have my own office, and every patient I would see had a pre-arranged appointment time. Not to say that it wasn't busy or that it wasn't hard work. It was just a more organized kind of busy, so a great deal less stress for me.

The next day, I was in home care. I also knew about this one in twenty minutes. Unfortunately, my opinion about this position was a great deal less favorable. To make matters worse, I still had an entire day to go through. We were on the road, so I couldn't exactly back out at that point. The woman who I was paired up with was great. She was very understanding and just allowed me to hang back. The first patient we went to see was bedbound. As soon as we walked into his house, I could feel the walls just closing in on me. That's the way I experience my anxiety, rather like claustrophobia. Everything begins to feel oppressive, like a great weight has been placed on me. I also have the sensation that it is becoming difficult to breath. Anyway,

I did manage to complete the day, but I knew that I wasn't coming back. The manager was a little taken aback when I told her this, because I had asked for two days of home care shadowing. I'm also sure that no one in her experience had ever turned down a job in home care before. They are highly sought-after positions. However, once I explained the situation, she totally understood.

I decided, obviously, that I would take the job in the clinic. First off, it was the perfect choice. It was also the only choice, since it was the only position that I had been able to find after months of searching. While it was quite heartening to finally have found a job that I could actually do, there were still a few hoops to jump through. All the players had to get together in one place: my employer, my old manager (from the ER), my new manager, the union, and a representative from ALMH. Trying to get everyone together was very much like trying to herd ducks. You find a time that works, but there's always the one person that can't make it. So, you find another time, and someone else is busy. And so on. Eventually, we hit upon a day that worked for everyone.

At that point, we all gathered together around a table, and we had a big discussion about how this was going to work. They couldn't just shove me into a line and hope for the best. There had to be a whole process, in case there were any problems. Just because I liked the job didn't mean that it was going to like me. I was the unknown factor here, and that had to be taken into account before we did anything else. They had to have some supports in place, such as ensuring that I had access to appropriate help if I started having a panic attack.

There were other details to work out as well, like who was going to pay me. That was certainly one of *my* biggest concerns. ALMH has the option to pay for the orientation period. This is done as an incentive so that managers will be more willing to take on someone with a disability. It also allowed me to still be in contact with ALMH during this time, in case I have need of them. After much discussion, it was decided that I would have an entire month of orientation. I liked that because I would not feel rushed to learn everything at once. I could just take my time getting settled. What I really didn't like was that I would continue to get paid by ALMH for the entire month. In other words, I was doing 100 percent of the work for 70 percent of the pay. That's a great arrangement for the hospital, but not so much for me. I would also have to continue paying out-of-pocket for my extended health, since I would still not be an official employee of the hospital. In truth, my ALMH benefits are not taxable, so it is probably close to what I would have been earning anyway. Still, it is a little less.

I did get my parking pass back, though.

...

Before I had even started in the new position, there was a great deal of homework to do. Most of the nurses who worked there had come from a surgical background. As a result, they all had a head start when it came to the pre-op patient teaching. I, on the other hand, had not been on a surgical floor since nursing school. That was a while ago. As a result, I had no idea what each of the surgeries really entailed. Because of this, I really wasn't sure what information the patients would need. I had a lot of reading to get through.

I was also required to take the new employee orientation again because I had been off for so long. That was an excruciating experience. I really hadn't forgotten all that much. Mostly, we went over the computer stuff, which was still familiar to me. There were a few new things that had been improved during the interim, and these changes did make it easier to use. However, the clinic used its own set of computerized forms, so it was mostly irrelevant to me anyway. Most of the people at the orientation were either new grads or they had come from other hospitals, so they needed to know all this stuff. I didn't. When they started to show us how to start IVs, my brain wanted to explode. That's when I decided to bail.

One positive thing did come out of the orientation. As I was the only returning employee, one of the women who was running the orientation asked if she could talk to me about the computer program we used. Apparently, she worked in a nearby hospital that was going to be using it soon. I agreed, and we arranged to meet up a week later. Well, when we did meet up, she really got an earful. I think she was expecting our talk to last about ten minutes. I kept her there for over an hour.

There were other considerations with this new job as well. For instance, I didn't own a single set of scrubs. In the ER, these had been provided for us. They were ratty looking, but we didn't have to pay for them, so we didn't care what they looked like. We also didn't have to worry about washing them. Now, I had to go shopping. Being a guy, I have always hated shopping, even before the anxiety came along. To make the experience even worse, you can just imagine how common guys' scrubs are. If you can't, the answer is not very. Also, the price of scrubs had gone up exponentially since I had last bought some. They were all designer floral prints, for $50 a pop. Some had frills. They were all tapered, as well.

I do not have hips. I do, however, have a belly. They were definitely not tapered for my figure. When I did find scrubs for men, they were completely devoid of pockets. For those of you that are unfamiliar, nurses absolutely love pockets. We want pockets everywhere. Big ones, small ones, ones that are shaped like scissors. It's all good. The perfect pair of scrubs would be made from nothing but pockets, all sewn together. Apparently, someone in the scrub making industry does not know this, or they have simply decided that this rule does not apply to men. They are wrong.

GUNFIRE IN THE DISTANCE

One thing that I have really become aware of in these past few months is just how much my confidence has taken a beating. I used to walk into new situations with a sense of confidence—not like I already knew everything, but still knowing that I could pick things up easily. I remember walking into my new job that day with a real sense of dread, which was another first for me. That first day, the feelings of uncertainty were so strong, I almost didn't make it through the door. I seriously wondered how long it would be before they realized what an idiot I was and sent me packing.

I have also realized that with the anxiety comes a genuine fear of new environments. They make me feel very uncomfortable, sometimes so much so that I can't even enter. Just recently, the gym near my house closed down for a month. Apparently, they do this once a year for maintenance. There is another gym close by, but I really don't like it. It's strange and foreign to me. I went twice but became so anxious about being there that I had to leave. Instead, I went out and bought some weights to use at home. I will return to my usual gym once it reopens. I will not be returning to the second one, however. I had that exact same sensation when I arrived at my new job.

This was not an auspicious beginning to my latest career endeavor. Still, I mustered up the courage and went inside.

I was placed with another nurse who was almost as new as I was. Funnily enough, she had also been hired there as a duty to accommodate. However, she had come from one of the surgical floors and had many years of experience. Right from the start, I was totally intimidated. I felt that I knew almost nothing by comparison.

...

There were four main components to my new job. First, we did the pre-op interviews for patients that were having more complicated surgeries (people who would be staying for a day or two post-op). The patients would usually come in a week or two before the big day. They would meet with someone from pharmacy in order to verify all the medications that they were taking at home. Then, they would come to see one of the nurses. Our job was to verify all their information, go over everything they would need to know about their surgery, answer any questions they had, and take note of any concerns that might require some follow-up.

The second thing we would do is to review patients charts before surgery. This was done mostly for the simpler procedures: things that would not require an overnight stay. We would ensure that all the information was correct and flag anything needing attention, just as we did for the bigger surgeries. The largest component of chart review days, however, was making sure that any tests the patient needed to have completed pre-op had actually been done. This was an easy thing to do with the other group, because they were right in the hospital already. We only had to give them the proper paperwork and direct them where to go for the tests. This group we did not meet in person, so that approach was not an option. Most of the time, the surgeons would order the tests. Sometimes, however, they would forget. More often, the patients would have the requisitions and just not bother to go. In these cases, we would have to phone the patients at home and nag them. It was really quite a simple concept. No tests, no surgery. Occasionally, it would take a few phone calls to get them going.

Our third task was to deal with the anesthetics appointments. On these days, they would meet with patients that we had flagged for various reasons. Most of the time, they would have a medical condition that could put them at risk during the surgery, such as diabetes (they take longer to heal), blood clotting disorders, and allergies to anesthetics. Occasionally, there would be questions about a medication that they were taking. On these days, our main function was to usher people in to see the anesthesiologist at the appropriate time. These were the only days that we would see patients who were grumpy. The nurses' appointment times were rigidly adhered to. I am sure you know how doctors can be, however. Sometimes the patients were kept waiting for quite a while, which would make them cranky. Occasionally, the anesthesiologist would have orders pertaining to the patient that had just been seen. It was also our job to enter these orders into the computer.

What I liked most about these days was that many of the anesthesiologists were very personable and approachable. They are also some of the smartest doctors around. It takes two more years of school, after becoming a doctor, to work in this specialty. Being very inquisitive myself, it was always good to be able to pick their brains on certain topics. It did take me a while to feel completely comfortable asking them things, though. As they rarely venture beyond the confines of the operating rooms, they were probably the only doctors in the hospital that I had never met before.

Our last duty was brand new. That is because there had already been a person doing it. She was going to be leaving her position, though. It was decided that, rather than hiring one person for the job, everyone would take turns doing it. This wasn't entirely a popular decision, as it involved coming in on evenings. By far, one of the best parts of this job was that it was straight nine-to-five (or eight-to-four in this case). No one was very keen on the idea of evening shifts.

This job was actually very similar to our first job but only involved patients coming in for day surgery (people who would go home post-op). It was a shortened and simpler process. Instead of coming in to see us, we would just phone them at home and ask them all the questions. That's why it had to be done in the evenings, so that people were more likely to be home.

The whole purpose of the work that we did was to avoid costly mistakes. Previously, patients would just show up on the day of their surgeries, and someone would have to go over all of this with them. That meant often having to delay surgeries because of things that the doctors had not been aware of beforehand. For instance, finding out that your patient is taking blood thinners. For obvious reasons, these have to be stopped a few days before surgery or else things can get messy. Even worse, sometimes things could be missed entirely, such as allergies that were not listed on the patient's chart. This could have devastating and sometimes even fatal results. As I am sure you can imagine, we generally prefer to avoid those types of outcomes.

Right from the beginning, the hardest part for me was remembering what pre-op instructions to give each patient. Most of the instructions could be applied to all surgeries, but some were different. For instance, the instructions specific to hip replacements differed significantly from those for an abdominal surgery. Sometimes, instructions would also differ for each surgeon. Trying to recall the specifics was quite a challenge for me when I first started. I did improve as time went on, thankfully. I read a great deal about all the different surgeries, in an effort to catch up to my co-workers. I listened closely to what everyone said. I pretty much memorized, word for word, the pre-op book that we sent home with patients. I took mounds of paper home with me every night to study.

I should also acknowledge that my ER background did end up having its advantages. After some time spent beating myself up for being dumb, I realized I had a wealth of knowledge that they didn't have because of my own background. For instance, I knew a little more than they did about medical conditions. One of the things we told patients to do pre-op was to load up on sugar the day before. The body requires energy to heal, so getting calories before surgery speeds recovery time. I was surprised, however, to learn that we did not do this for our diabetic patients. Most of the people I talked to did not understand my concerns. After all, everyone knows that diabetics have to avoid sugar. Well, because I have a greater understanding of diabetes, I was able to make a good case. I won't go into all the technical details for you, so you won't be bored. Suffice it to say that too much sugar is not the problem with diabetics. *Lack* of insulin is. One of the most persistent myths among nurses is that diabetes is all about sugar. The reality is that diabetics are slower to heal, so they might even benefit more from loading up on sugar before surgery, as long as they also receive a corresponding dose of insulin. Because of my concerns, this was one of the topics that I brought up with the anesthesiologist. I was told that it was already in the works. They just needed a proper protocol in place for close monitoring of diabetic patients post-op, because their sugar levels still need to be controlled. This protocol had not been developed yet. See, I told you they know everything.

For the first week, I basically just followed people around, listening to how they would conduct the interviews. The first week was also when I got my first nasty surprise. There was something wrong with the lock on the bathroom door, so a maintenance guy was sent down to fix it. I am not sure what exactly was wrong with it, but they worked on that door for the entire day.

I could have built an entirely new bathroom in that amount of time. Being very sensitive to noise, the constant buzzing of saws and drills for my entire shift had me feeling very stressed out when I finally went home. My quiet little corner of the hospital had been invaded, and I was not at all pleased about it. It took several hours of silence before I was able to calm down.

The next day, thankfully, things went back to normal. All was quiet again.

As time progressed, I did start to feel more knowledgeable about the surgical stuff. I started doing the interviews with the patients myself, though I was super slow at first. I liked talking to the patients, but chatting is a bit of a time waster, especially with some of the older folks. They love to talk. We were allotted forty-five minutes per patient, so keeping a steady pace was essential. Still, I believe that patients who feel like they have been listened to and acknowledged are going to be far more satisfied with their overall experience than patients who don't. Here's the thing. Most people think that hospitals get sued when the staff do something wrong. Often, that is not actually the case. We really get sued over how patients and families perceive the events. Statistically, we are at greater risk of litigation from what we don't do, rather than from what we do. Failing to order a test that the patient felt was needed is more likely to end up in court than making an error. Talking to patients and making them feel valued is a huge part of that perception, with better experiences coming from more interaction with staff, not less. It also gives the patients more time to ask questions. Increased knowledge leads to decreased fear, which also improves outcomes. It gives the staff more time to ensure that instructions are understood, as well. This makes patients more likely to follow directions, which leads to faster recovery times. There was talk, when I left, of taking the interviews down to thirty minutes. This was an idea that I was definitely not in favor of.

One thing that really interested me was listening to how each nurse conducted their interviews. There were a few nurses who worked there, and each had their own style. Some were more detail oriented than others. Some just talked to the patients, using a more conversational and less structured approach. I watched for what I thought worked well and what didn't. As time passed, this gave me a great base for developing my own style. I seemed to fit somewhere in the middle.

With practice, I had really improved. I still forgot things, but they weren't the big things anymore. It also wasn't as often. The woman who was doing most of my orientation relied heavily on a scripted interview, and I could see her face scrunch up whenever I missed something. Usually, I could catch what I had forgotten and throw it in later.

I also got to spend some time with one of the pharmacy techs. I got to watch one of her interviews, and it provided me with a good perspective on what they looked for. There is a unique style to the way in which the pharmacy techs conduct their interviews. I know very well how difficult their job is because I have also had to get the same information on occasion. Asking patients about their medications is often like pulling teeth. As a result, they have to really get in there and pry the information out. One thing I have found throughout my nursing career is just how difficult it can be to get an accurate medication history from people. Some have no idea what they are taking. They will tell you how they take a little red one and a large yellow one. Others will include only prescription medications, forgetting about the aspirin they take every morning. Vitamins are frequently left out because people tend to think of them as benign. In fact, vitamins can often interact with some medications. For instance, certain vitamins can affect how well blood thinners work. They can also have effects all on their own. I have seen quite a few niacin (one of the B vitamins) overdoses in my time. Their faces go all red.

Then, there are the people who just plain lie. They don't want to tell you about the pot that they smoke daily or the cocaine they used last night. For starters, the nurses don't care what you do. We're not cops. We are certainly not there to get you into trouble or to judge you. We really do *need* to know, however. Street drugs can have deadly side effects, especially when mixed with drugs that we might have to give you. And we are very likely going to find out anyway. That's what all those blood and urine tests are for. We don't test your pee because we're bored. Then, once we do find out, we're very likely to think you're an idiot for lying to us. That will get you off to a very bad start, I guarantee you. So just be honest.

I had a patient once who almost died because of a situation like this. We couldn't figure out what was wrong with him, and everyone with him swore to us that he would never touch drugs. He ended up in the ICU. Once he recovered, it came out that it *was* drug related. Had we known the true history, we probably could have treated him much faster.

Another thing I often find is just how ignorant people are about what their medications actually do. So many times, I'll see their medication list and have this conversation:

Me: "Oh, I see you are on a pill for high blood pressure. Do you have hypertension?"

Them: "Not since I started taking the pills."

Me: Face palm.

Just because you are taking the pills does not mean that the condition has gone away. Hint: if it had, you wouldn't need to take the pills anymore.

I bet that there's at least a few people reading this who do the exact same thing. They are probably scowling at me right now.

During my training, I also spent two afternoons with the woman who was doing the evening shifts at that time. Luckily, it wasn't that different from what I was already doing. Besides, almost no one ever seemed to be home, so we didn't have to talk a lot anyway. At least, that was my experience.

Another aspect of the job that I really appreciated was being able to provide feedback. The department was in the middle of revising the written materials that were provided to patients, and I was given the opportunity to have a say. Not much of a say because I was brand new of course. Besides, I don't think I really had much to add at that point. There were also some big schedule changes that were going to be happening, so the whole staff got together and talked about what that would look like.

My big issue, probably because of my ER background, was the appalling lack of security that we had been provided. Our offices were located in a back hallway, out of view. Most of our patients were polite, but that doesn't mean that all of them were going to be. Not to mention that anyone else could easily have wandered back there. If someone had decided to go at one of the staff, it might have gone completely unnoticed until it was all over. Around that time, a similar incident had happened at another hospital. No one had realized what was going on and the nurse had been trapped for half an hour. Because of this, I really pushed for having panic buttons installed in all the rooms. Then, in the event that a situation did get out of hand, we would at least be able to call for help. I'm not sure if they ever did install them after I left.

All in all, things seemed to be progressing quite well, and I was really enjoying my new position. By the third week, I was even spending some time on my own, doing the interviews without supervision. Of course, this is when I started to have problems. In truth, I had never fully gotten past the feelings that I had experienced on the very first day. I am certain that this contributed to what happened next.

The first incident occurred early one afternoon. I was doing chart reviews when I heard someone yelling at the unit clerk's desk. When I went out, a woman was sitting in front of the desk, and she was insisting that she needed some help right away. It was obvious that she had confused our area with the emergency department. The poor unit clerk was trying her best to explain that this was the wrong place, but the woman continued to insist that she be helped immediately. It was obvious that the situation was escalating, until the woman just exploded. Believing that this was very likely going to end in violence, I quickly intervened. I grabbed a wheelchair, had the woman take a seat, and proceeded to wheel her up to the ER. Once there, I dropped her off at the triage desk and returned to my office.

This event strongly impacted me. In my head, I was right back in the ER again. For the rest of the day, I was incredibly anxious. I very nearly had another panic attack. This event had me so flustered that I completely screwed up the chart review. I missed an entire two days' worth of charts. I also had a nightmare about the event that night. It was the first time that I had felt genuinely frightened at my new job. I began to spiral downward once again.

Toward the end of the third week, there was yet another triggering event. There were three code blues in the emergency department that morning, all about five minutes apart. All code blues get called overhead throughout the hospital. Because of this, I had to listen to the announcements each time. Back-to-back. My heart was just pounding after the last one. I was so wired that I can't even recall the rest of the day.

Not only did hearing that make me feel very anxious, but I also felt more than a little depressed. There is a part of me that still mourns for my old life, I guess. As a result, not being able to help with the code blues weighs on my emotions just as strongly. I feel that I am missing out somehow. It's a very keen sense of loss. I don't know if that will make sense to you or not.

More nightmares. Not sleeping. Not being able to focus again. I began to suffer from wicked heartburn every day. I was falling apart all over again. I tried very hard to hold it together, but nothing seemed to be working. I started missing important questions in my interviews, as well. Not the harder stuff, but the easy to remember stuff. I don't think that I was able to eat for three days straight.

A few nights later, I ended up in the ER having another panic attack. Just imagine that for a moment. I'm having a panic attack, and my only recourse for help is to go to the very place that caused my panic attacks in the first place. If it hadn't been happening to me, my dark sense of humor probably would have delighted in the irony of it all.

This is not the first time I have been into the ER with symptoms of anxiety. It will definitely not be the last. I am fortunate that my co-workers are aware of the situation. I get to sit in one of the quiet rooms for a few hours until the feeling of panic goes away. On this particular occasion, I think my heart rate was about 130 when I first arrived.

Many people found it hard to understand what was going on with me. After all, this seemed like the perfect job. I had a few friends ask me how *they* could get a job there. The way that I explained it to people was like this: It was like staying at a five-star hotel, but still being able to hear the sound of gunfire in the distance. The environment was still too similar for me to manage.

In the end, I had to leave that position. Yet again, I found myself without a job. I felt horrible, as if I had let people down. I know that they took a risk in hiring me. If not for the duty to accommodate, I doubt if I ever would have gotten a job there. It is such a good place to work, I imagine the only way they ever have an opening is if someone dies or retires. As a result, it was even harder for me to just drop out like that. In the end, I guess that I didn't really have a choice in the matter.

I BROKE IT AGAIN

So here I am, sitting at home once again. I have become even more reclusive and agoraphobic now, so I don't venture outside very much. I do still go out to the gym, or at least I did until it closed for the month. I have recently started to do some volunteer work as well. I see my therapist once a month. That's about it. Most of the time I stay in my little hidey-hole and watch the world outside go by.

At least no one has tried to take back my parking pass yet.

Of course, what fun would life be without some sort of weirdness from ALMH. Once again, I find that the rules are getting in my way. When you first apply for benefits, NATH takes you through steps one to ten. They get you help and anything else you might need to go back to your old job. Once that is no longer an option, they transfer you over to ALMH, who then takes you through steps eleven and twelve. The problem now is that I currently find myself back at step one. The experiences I had during my time at the new job have been a huge setback. They have brought on a full relapse of the PTSD. I can't even contemplate going back to work again at this point. I need full-time therapy again. ALMH, however, can only take me back as far as step eleven. Their purpose is to find me a new position, whether I am ready for one or not. They did get me back in to see the therapist, as I mentioned, but it's nowhere near as often as last time.

To use the broken leg analogy again, it's as if I have broken my leg a second time. Meanwhile, ALMH is busy telling me that they have already fixed my leg, so everything is great now. It's done. They can't seem to grasp the fact that I am right back where I started, emotionally.

It doesn't really matter what jobs are available at this point. It could be the calmest environment ever, and it would not matter one little bit. That's because I am never calm. The anxiety and fear are always there.

My biggest concern is that I cannot try and fail again. Having PTSD is a little like getting a concussion. Once you have had one, it's that much easier to get another one. The third one is even easier than that, and each successive one becomes more damaging as well. If I am put into a new position and it goes sideways again, I may just come out of this a total emotional basket case. That doesn't really work for me, as I am sure you will understand. It's not that I don't want to go back to work. I am pretty damn keen on it, actually. I want to do it right, though. If I go back too early, we're just going to end up right back where we started from. We could even end up with my mood becoming much worse. This is my brain they are playing with.

To be honest, if I can't even go to a new gym, what possible chance do I have at a new job?

Thankfully, everyone is away on vacation right now, so I have bought myself some time. It's hard to call anyone when they aren't there. For now, I'll just keep my head down and try not to draw any attention to myself.

My goal right now is to finish this book and become a famous writer. Then I can just avoid the whole mess altogether. Please, if you are reading this book, buy some copies for your friends as well.

There are so many things that have changed in my life. I used to be spontaneous and carefree. Now, everything takes so much planning. I can't just go out anymore. Now, I must take precautions when I have to go somewhere. If I know it is going to be crowded, I either have to find someone to go with or I take earplugs so that I can't hear the noise. One evening recently, I was just so sick of being cooped up that I forced myself to go to a nearby street market. I started to feel anxious from the minute I arrived. There was a lot going on, and there were people everywhere. Still, I was managing to keep it under control with the help of my earplugs. Then, some young woman who was dancing through the crowd came up to me and grabbed my hand. She smiled at me like we were the best of friends, but I had never laid eyes on her in my life. I suspect she may have been more than a little high. Now, most guys my age might be a little flattered after such an experience. At the very least, many people would see it as harmless. Not me. I was totally freaked out and had to leave immediately. Someone had deliberately entered my bubble. I haven't been back to the market since then.

I have also become a list person. I used to hate list people, I used to make fun of them. Now, every little thing has to be written down. I carry a notebook with me at all times, and I am constantly planning out my every step in there. Lists for what I have to do today, lists for what I need to bring. God help me if I am going away somewhere. Last month, I went camping with my sister. It was all very exciting, because I have never been car camping before. Usually, I like to go deep into the woods, away from everything. Well, not only did I have lists galore, but I had everything packed and organized about a week beforehand. If you are a list person, I humbly apologize for any of the rude things I may have said about you in the past. Truly, I joke about this, but there is a serious side. The lists are really all about control, and that need is completely new to me. I can't be spontaneous anymore because the anxiety just won't allow it.

One really odd change is that I now hate having the covers on me as I sleep. I used to be a cocooner. I would wrap myself up in a big, fluffy comforter every night. All my girlfriends over the years will tell you what a blanket hog I used to be. Now, I have the comforter pushed to the side of the bed most nights. Even a sheet makes me feel too warm. At most, I will cover up my midsection if I get cold. I puzzled over this for some time as it didn't seem to make any logical sense. After all, what do blankets have to do with my post-traumatic stress. Well, it turns out that being cooler at night helps the body to regulate cortisol levels. That's one of the stress hormones. Without even being consciously aware of it, my body was responding to the anxiety. As a nurse, I found that rather interesting.

I also had to double the dosage of all my medications. At least that helps a little. The nightmares have subsided again, but they haven't gone away completely. I also asked my doctor for some sleeping pills, just so that I am able to get a good night's rest every so often. I think she is worried that I might start taking them every night and become addicted, because she gave me a very stern warning. No worries there. I love the sleep, but I wake up with the most awful taste in my mouth. It's as if I have been chewing on an eraser for the entire night. I will be using them sparingly, trust me.

She also added a new medication that makes me feel pretty dopey sometimes.

With the increased dosages, I have really noticed a problem with constipation. Some days, it can get downright unpleasant. Fortunately, I have also recently discovered bran muffins.

When I say that I am anxious all the time, I really mean it. My anxiety sits at about a three out of ten now. It gets worse if there is something going on around me that is triggering. Some of the things that ramp it up are loud noises, sudden noises, sirens going by, crowds, new places, anything that "bings," anyone who looks sick in public, anything to do with hospitals on TV, being in the hospital, talking to anyone I don't know, hearing a child cry, and any sudden movements near me. I am sure that I have forgotten a few.

For some reason, the anxiety always gets stronger during the evenings. I have no idea why.

My sister and I have this running chicken joke. Her ring tone on my phone used to be a singing chicken. I had to change it because every time she called me, I just about had a heart attack.

There is one thing that I am very curious about these days. I have heard that MDMA (Ecstasy) has been showing great promise as a treatment for PTSD. Unfortunately, it's unlikely to be approved before 2022. I would just go downtown and buy some if it weren't for all the damn fentanyl around these days.

When ALMHagreed to give me more therapy sessions, I was able to go back to see the same guy, so that made me happy. He seemed almost disappointed to see me again, like we should have done better the first time. We don't do the tapping thing anymore. Now we just talk. It feels good just to be able to unburden sometimes, and he's a very good listener. I'm not entirely certain what I am looking for this time, though. Last time we did this, I was looking for a cure. Now, I think I would just like to have some sense of normalcy in my life. At the very least, reducing the symptoms would give me some functionality again. Not jumping six feet into the air every time I hear a loud noise would be really nice too.

Believe it or not, I would still one day like to return to the ER. It is the whole reason I became a nurse in the first place. I recognize, however, that I can't go back to it as it is right now. I have many changes to make within myself, but the system needs to be very different as well. Right now, conditions there are exactly the same as when I left. That place may never get any better. I may never be able to work there again, and that is a possibility I need to accept.

I have started doing some volunteer work with the SPCA, just to keep myself busy. My sister had suggested this as a possibility. She was concerned about my growing isolation and thought that this might be a great way to meet people. Truth is, if I had wanted to meet people, I wouldn't have volunteered at the SPCA. I am much more interested in meeting some cats and dogs. When I am there, I spend most of my time helping the paid staff to keep the place clean. I do the laundry and the dishes for them. I mostly keep to myself when I am there. I still don't do people very well, so I just do my own thing. I do love the kittens, but that can be hit and miss. One week there were only two cats there. The cats also have a tendency to sleep for most of the day, which is when I am there. Lazy bastards. Next week, I am going for an orientation in the dog section, and I am looking forward to spending some time with them as well.

The main problem with volunteering at the SPCA is that I want to take all the animals home at the end of every shift. Unfortunately, my apartment building doesn't allowed pets. I could push it if I really wanted to. I would be eligible for a therapy animal, due to the anxiety. No one can refuse to allow a therapy animal. When I asked the building manager about it, she did not look very pleased, and I decided that it wasn't the hill I wanted to die on. They might not be able to kick me out for that, but I'm sure they could find some other reason if they wanted to.

Instead, I got myself some therapy gerbils, which are probably the worst therapy animals ever. They are even more neurotic than I am.

I also bought myself a teddy bear on the advice of my therapist. Apparently, it can work much like a therapy animal for people who aren't allowed to have pets. It's not as crazy as it sounds. In the hospital, they give heart patients stuffed hearts to go home with. They're supposed to give it a big hug whenever they get anxious or stressed, and it is supposed to soothe them. I will see if it does the same for me.

On my first day at the SPCA, I noticed that I had a very similar reaction to going in as I had at my previous job. That fear of failure again. This is a volunteer job, so I am sure they are just glad to have me. Still, that same fear was there.

The depression that I feel on some days is almost crippling. I just feel like crying for the entire day. This comes on even stronger after a panic attack. It feels like failure to me, as if I should be able to control my anxiety. I have become fantastic at wallowing. No one can do self-pity like I can these days. Sometimes, all I can seem to think about is what a big loser I have become.

That pretty much sums up my life these days. Appointments galore. The SPCA. The gym. Writing. Occasionally sleeping. That's it. Not very exciting, I know, but for now that's a good thing.

During this time, I have been looking into alternatives. One idea I had was to become a nursing instructor. For that, however, I would need to get my master's degree. In nursing, there are several different graduate programs to choose from. Most of them are all theory, which doesn't appeal to me in the least. That would be like going back to nursing school, and I would gouge my own eyes out before going through that again. There is one option that I am interested in: the nurse practitioner program. A nurse practitioner is an advanced nursing specialty. They are kind of like a nurse/doctor hybrid. The program is much more technical, which I would definitely enjoy. The problem is that it's a very expensive program to take.

I also looked into the possibility of working with the nursing students without getting my degree. When I asked, the university told me that all I would be able to do without getting a master's degree is work with the students during their clinical placements. That would entail being in the hospital, so that's a no go. I doubt it would instill confidence if the instructor was hiding under the desk all day.

My last option is to leave nursing altogether. There is a program at the university to become a regular teacher. Because I already have a bachelor's degree, there is a consolidated course that only takes eighteen months. That would be pretty sweet. It's also a great deal less expensive.

Unfortunately, ALMH is not on board with any of these ideas. They want me back at work. Somehow, it makes more sense to keep trying the same thing over and over, rather than attempt something different.

Besides, even going back to school is probably not an option at this point. I have to see at least some improvement first.

I have also been trying very hard to get the top brass out here to adopt a PTSD prevention strategy. So far, everyone seems very excited by the whole idea. Unfortunately, no one wants to actually *do* anything about it. I leave messages for people who call me back six months later or not at all. So far, no one even seems to know for sure who would be in charge of such a thing. When I do manage to reach people, they usually tell me ten other people that I have to call instead of them. My enthusiasm for this project has definitely waned over time. There's only so long that a person can bang their head against a brick wall.

The sad thing is that nursing is falling behind the times. The military has recognized the problem for years. Some time ago, a psychiatrist designed an entire program for the paramedics. For nurses, it's barely even begun to be recognized as an issue. When we do talk about it, it's presented as an ER or ICU problem. Certainly, critical care nurses are more susceptible, but only because we are exposed to more. All nurses are at risk, especially with conditions in the hospitals the way they are now. No one seems to be in any particular rush to do anything about it, however.

Recently, a few more of my co-workers have developed the same symptoms. This makes me incredibly angry. Despite my efforts, two years have passed by and nothing has changed.

I do try to spread my message as often as possible, though. I have given talks at some of the nursing schools. I talk to my colleagues as often as I can to remind them about self-care and to share their stories with others. I also did an interview for an article that my union put out.

One of the talks I gave was at my old nursing school. My big message is disclosure. If something happens, don't stuff it down. Tell people about it. Yell it out at the top of your lungs before it eats you alive. I am told that the message really hit home. It had such a great effect, in fact, that the instructors spent the entire rest of the day meeting with individual students. All of them wanted to share. When I do speak, I try to keep the message positive as well. The last thing I want to do is scare away new nurses. We need them desperately. My goal is to see them last in this profession, so I want to provide them with some strategies that will help them to succeed. The most important strategy of all is honesty.

The local university wouldn't even let me talk to their students. Apparently, everything is fine in nursing, and they don't want me to be bringing up any problems. We shall see how that strategy works out for them.

I thought that the article was a big win as well. It really shone a light on what nurses actually go through in a day. In particular, the article used my story to illustrate just how much stress we face during a shift and how devastating the consequences can be when that stress is not properly managed afterwards. Because of the campaign that the article was a part of, we now have it mandated that ER nurses can claim for PTSD without having to go through all the bureaucracy. Our claims are now rushed through, and it is now just assumed to be job related. Next on the agenda is to get that policy extended to all nurses. I say, go even further with it. Witnessing traumatic events can happen on any job and that needs to be recognized.

There was one thing that really upset me about helping with the article, however. No one bothered to tell me when it was published. Instead, I had a friend call one evening to tell me that they had just read it. They thought it was great. Meanwhile, I'm in a total panic. I ended up scrambling around town in the late evening, trying to find someone who still had a copy of the newspaper it was in. Understandably, I really wanted to save it. I did manage to find the last copy in town, after going to every store within ten miles of my house.

I also wrote my own article. Unfortunately, no one has seemed very interested in it. Apparently, I am a little too harsh with my employer and with NATH. No one wants a lawsuit. I did find one magazine that wanted to publish it, but they appear to have vanished from the earth. Now I have this book instead. And they thought that the article was too harsh...

And so, life continues. This is by no means the end of my story, but I did have to stop at some point. Had I not, this book could well have gone on forever. In any case, I hope that you have enjoyed my tale.

One final thing, speaking of NATH. Today was payday. I got up this morning expecting to go grocery shopping and pay some bills. I logged in to my account and no money. I thought to myself that perhaps it just hadn't gone through yet. Hours later, still no money. Now I am getting anxious (or more anxious, to be precise). I called them but got voicemail instead. There's a number to call, though, if my problem is urgent. I'm pretty sure that this qualifies. Oh, but the urgent call number goes to voicemail as well. Two more calls and I still wasn't getting an actual person. I called my bank, just to make sure it's not a problem on their end. Nope, everything's fine there. Finally, I managed to get a worker on the phone. She had no idea what is going on, so she said she will attempt to find *my* worker and then phone me back. She did a few hours later. Turns out that the check is waiting, but someone forgot to authorize it, so it's stuck in a computer somewhere. They forgot? That's kind of a big oops, or at least it is for me. Then she informed me that the check has now been authorized and should be deposited into my account within three business days. "So sorry." That's ok. It's not like I need the money, right? Thank god for Mastercard. It's no wonder I have anxiety.

FINAL WORDS

Y ou don't have to read this part if you don't want too. If you have enjoyed the story, that is all I really want. If you are interested in hearing some of my ideas about possible solutions, then read on.

This is where we get down to business. I would be very disappointed if all anyone took from my story is a sense of doom. The point of writing this book was not to complain about a broken system. My purpose was to point out the flaws in the system so that they can be fixed. There is hope to be found here. My story need not be the template for those that follow.

Stress is not a minor problem. It is becoming an epidemic in health care, and the numbers are alarming. One article that I have seen often cited found that 14 percent of nurses exhibit some or all of the symptoms of PTSD. That is four times higher than the general population. Now, this does not mean that they have PTSD, only that they are on the spectrum (they have some of the symptoms, but not enough for an official diagnosis). In critical care areas such as ICU, that number jumps to 25 percent. ER nurses lead the way with 33 percent (Hood).

It is not enough to improve the way we respond to PTSD in the workplace. We must also take steps to prevent it. Mental health safety needs to be given the same level of consideration as physical safety or nothing will ever change. What follows are just some ideas that I have come up with that will begin to move us in the right direction.

First, I would really like to see mandatory debriefing sessions after *every* critical incident. This doesn't mean that everyone has to come. You can't force people, after all. I do believe, however, that the employer should have to make one available. Then people can come if they wish. I do think that staff should be strongly encouraged to attend.

I also believe that there should be people trained in running the debriefs right in the hospital. They should also be nurses or other health care professionals. We need people who speak our language and who know what our work is like. People who won't tell us to drink some more water. These are called peer debriefers, and they should respond whenever a code is called within the hospital. We already do this with other services. When the person is needed, they get coverage for the time they are gone from their post. After the code (or other critical incident) is finished, they would be able to run a debrief right in the moment, rather than waiting a few days until someone is available.

There also needs to be a great deal of staff education on appropriate stress management. Our job is very hard. We spend every single day with people who are having the worst day of their lives. To see what we do and think that we won't be touched by it is ludicrous. Stuffing it down does not work. There has been a rise in suicide rates for health care workers over the last few years. The few studies that have been done show that stress and burnout are rampant in the industry. This is true across the board, in every area. To combat this, we need to talk. We should be talking to each other, to our significant others, to our loved ones. If it helps, tell the guy sitting next to you on the bus. Whatever it takes. We don't need to provide details. It's enough just to say, "Hey, I've had a really horrible day."

One idea that I try to push forward is what I call the "crap buddy." This involves making a pact with someone. Both people promise that whatever happens, the other one will always be ready to listen without judgement. "I made a mistake today." "This horrible thing happened." "This situation made me feel really uncomfortable." Whatever. The point is, this is the one person that you can say anything to.

Another idea that I had was to actually rotate nurses out of critical care areas, just like they do with soldiers. Six months in, six months out. That sort of idea. Perhaps a job share program with home care nurses or in other areas. I imagine that many of my fellow nurses would hate this, but I believe it would go a long way toward preventing PTSD.

Also, we need to know what the signs of stress, burnout, and PTSD are. I didn't have any idea what was happening to me at first. We need to post this information everywhere. We need to tell nurses and doctors what to watch for in themselves, and we need to be watching out for the signs in each other as well. If we see someone struggling, we can identify the problem if we are given the right tools. We can then support that person in finding the help that they need. Part of this could be online screening tools that people could use, confidentially. This would make them both available and easily accessible to all.

A huge part of this will be destigmatizing mental health problems in our industry. People need to know that it is ok to be struggling or they will never seek help. It is not a failure, and it is not a sign of weakness. Given what we face on a day-to-day basis, it's called being human.

We need to make information on how to get help readily available. I went through the early days of my illness feeling around in the dark. That approach makes healing harder and is counterproductive in the long run. There needs to be a process, and health care workers need to know what that process is.

Sick days. We always see sick days as being for physical injuries or illnesses. "My stomach is upset, so I won't be in today." Mental health days are important as well, and we need to allow for that. In fact, these should be encouraged, within reason of course. Instead, we applaud people who never call in sick, and people who call in sick frequently get reprimanded. Balance is the key. No one should be calling in sick every other day, but no one should be coming in when they are already stressed out either.

NATH also needs to look at their policies. There should be be policies in place that are specific to mental health injuries. Help needs to be provided immediately for those in crisis. Yes, we have that available through our work already, but that help is both limited in scope and less than sufficient in length. It is meant to deal with simpler problems and lacks the capacity for immediately aiding those with real emotional trauma.

There should also be more realistic expectations around returning to work. Putting people right back into the same environment is probably not the best way to ensure success. Having realistic alternatives is a way to improve outcomes for people, ensuring that they have a position that will not be taxing on them emotionally. Speeding up the process will help with this. I truly believe that the longer I have had to wait, the more entrenched my anxiety becomes. Not having a job and not having contact with the outside world for so long decreases my chances of making a meaningful recovery. I have also lost confidence in myself over time, which only makes the entire situation worse. We need to learn from this so that it can be prevented next time.

Perhaps the most important thing is that we must take a look at workload. We need limits, and those limits have to be policy! They should be literally written in stone. A nurse who is overwhelmed is a nurse who is destined for some type of emotional injury. It becomes a matter of when, not if. Policies around workload limits not only benefit staff, but they are *cheaper* in the long run. Constantly working overtime, having to replace and retrain staff, paying out sick time. These are all huge inefficiencies, and they can be easily solved by increasing baseline staff. I am a highly trained professional. My employer has invested a great deal of time and money in me so that I could become a great nurse. Now, I sit at home instead.

Lastly, we need to put an end to the toxic workplace culture that blames health care workers for the shortcomings in the system. We are neither stupid nor lazy, and we need that to be recognized by both administrators and the public at large. Bullying needs to become unacceptable, especially from our peers and our superiors. There are no excuses for this anymore.

Anyway, that's just my two cents.

ACKNOWLEDGMENTS

To all the people that I have worked with over the years, you are an inspiration. Each of you has helped to shape my own practice, in your own way. Each and every one of you is a true hero.

To all those who have helped me in the writing of this book, I say a heartfelt thank-you. I also apologize profusely.

To coffee, for making my life so much better. This book might have taken far longer to write without you.

To my sister, who has kept me moving forward. To Michelle, for your endless enthusiasm and for putting up with my endless nagging.

To the health care system. Without your endless, maddening bureaucracy, I would never have been inspired to write this book.

To Storm Large and Tilda Shalof, whose memoirs inspired me to write mine.

Lastly, to all of the patients I have had over the years, behave yourselves. I am quite sure that every last one of you never wants to see me again (in a professional capacity, at least).

WORKS CITED

Hood, MAJ Deborah A. "PTSD in Nurses." *Elite Learning*, 4 Feb. 2011, www.elitecme.com/resource-center/nursing/ptsd-in-nurses/.

Schnell, Scott, et al. "The 1-Year Mortality of Patients Treated in a Hip Fracture Program for Elders." *Geriatric Orthopaedic Surgery & Rehabilitation*, vol. 1, no. 1, 2010, pp. 6-14, doi:10.1177/2151458510378105.

Schwartz, J. (2013). *Rachel Naomi Remen – Addiction & Recovery News*. [online] Addiction & Recovery News. Available at: https://addictionan-drecoverynews.wordpress.com/tag/rachel-naomi-remen/ [Accessed 25 Oct. 2019].

CPSIA information can be obtained
at www.ICGtesting.com
Printed in the USA
LVHW111400150822
725980LV00014B/256/J